QUICK GUIDE TO
Cardiopulmonary Care

EDITOR

Peter R. Lichtenthal, M.D.

Chief, Cardiovascular Anesthesia
Northwestern Memorial Hospital
Northwestern University
Chicago, Illinois

Table of Contents

Table of Contents continued on page iii

Functional Anatomy

For hemodynamic monitoring purposes, the right and left heart are differentiated as to function, structure and pressure generation. The pulmonary capillary bed lies between the right and left heart. The capillary bed is a compliant system with a high capacity to sequester blood.

The circulatory system consists of two circuits in a series: pulmonic circulation, which is a low-pressure system with low resistance to blood flow; and the systemic circulation, which is a high-pressure system with high resistance to blood flow.

RIGHT AND LEFT HEART DIFFERENCES

Right Heart	Left Heart
Receives deoxygenated blood	Receives oxygenated blood
Low pressure system	High pressure system
Volume pump	Pressure pump
RV thin and crescent shape	LV thick and conical shape
Coronary perfusion biphasic	Coronary perfusion during diastole

ANATOMICAL STRUCTURES

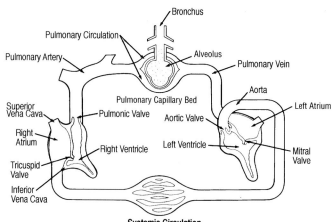

Systemic Circulation

Coronary Arteries and Veins

The two major branches of the coronary arteries arise from each side of the aortic root. Each coronary artery lies in the atrioventricular sulcus and is protected by a layer of adipose tissue.

Major Branches	Areas Supplied
Right Coronary Artery (RCA)	Sinus Node 55%, AV Node 90%, Bundle of His (90%) RA, RV free wall Portion of IVS
Posterior Descending Branch (Provided by RCA 80%)	Posterior wall of LV Portion of IVS
Left Main Coronary Artery Bifurcates:	
Left Anterior Descending (LAD)	Left anterior wall Anterior portion of IVS Portion of right ventricle
Left Circumflex (Provided by Posterior Branch 20%)	Sinus node 45%, LA
	Lateral wall of LV

Coronary Veins	Location Drains Into
Thebesian Veins	Directly into R & L ventricles
Great Cardiac Vein	Coronary sinus in the RA
Anterior Cardiac Veins	RV

CORONARY ARTERIES

Blood is supplied to heart tissues by branches of the coronary arteries.

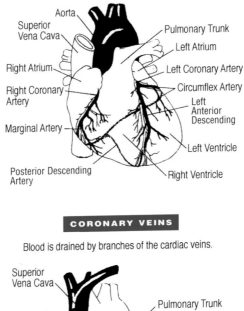

Aorta
Superior Vena Cava
Right Atrium
Right Coronary Artery
Marginal Artery
Posterior Descending Artery

Pulmonary Trunk
Left Atrium
Left Coronary Artery
Circumflex Artery
Left Anterior Descending
Left Ventricle
Right Ventricle

CORONARY VEINS

Blood is drained by branches of the cardiac veins.

Superior Vena Cava
Aorta
Right Atrium
Anterior Cardiac Vein
Small Cardiac Vein
Inferior Vena Cava

Pulmonary Trunk
Left Atrium
Left Ventricle
Right Ventricle
Middle Cardiac Vein

Cardiac Cycle: Electrical Correlation to Mechanical

Electrical cardiac cycle occurs prior to mechanical cardiac cycle. Atrial depolarization begins from the SA node. This current is then transmitted throughout the ventricles. Following the wave of depolarization, muscle fibers contract, which produces systole.

The next electrical activity is repolarization which results in the relaxation of the muscle fibers and produces diastole. The time difference between the electrical and mechanical activity is called electro-mechanical coupling, or the excitation-contraction phase. A simultaneous recording of the ECG and pressure tracing will show the electrical wave before the mechanical wave.

ELECTRICAL - MECHANICAL CARDIAC CYCLE

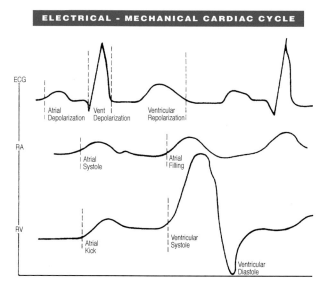

Mechanical Cardiac Cycle Phases

SYSTOLE

Isovolumetric Phase
Follows QRS of ECG
All valves are closed
Majority of oxygen consumed

Rapid Ventricular Ejection
Occurs during ST segment
80% to 85% of blood volume ejected

Reduced Ventricular Ejection
Occurs during "T" wave
Atria are in diastole
Produces "v" wave in atrial tracing

DIASTOLE

Isovolumetric Relaxation
Follows "T" wave
All valves closed
Ventricular pressure declines further
Ends in the ventricular "diastolic dip"

Rapid Ventricular Filling
AV valves open
Approximately two-thirds of blood volume goes into ventricle

Slow Filling Phase: End-Diastole
"Atrial Kick"
Follows "P" wave during sinus rhythms
Atrial systole occurs
Produces "a" wave on atrial tracings
Remaining volume goes into ventricle

Coronary Artery Perfusion

Coronary artery perfusion for the left ventricle occurs primarily during diastole. The increase in ventricular wall stress during systole increases resistance to such an extent that there is very little blood flow into the endocardium. During diastole there is less wall tension so a pressure gradient occurs that promotes blood flow through the left coronary arteries. The right ventricle has less muscle mass, therefore less wall stress during systole, so that due to less resistance more blood flows through the right coronary artery during systole. Optimal RV performance depends in part on this biphasic perfusion. There must be adequate diastolic pressure in the aortic root for both coronary arteries to be perfused.

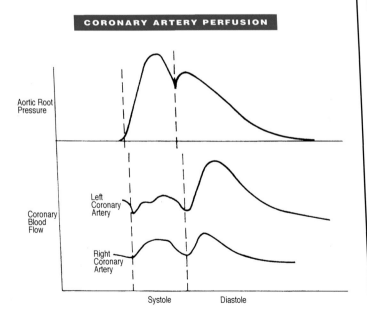

CORONARY ARTERY PERFUSION

Aortic Root Pressure

Coronary Blood Flow

Left Coronary Artery

Right Coronary Artery

Systole   Diastole

Swan-Ganz Catheter Port Locations and Functions

LOCATION	COLOR	FUNCTION
Distal	Yellow	Monitors PA pressures
Proximal	Blue	Monitors RA pressures, used for cardiac output injectate fluid
Balloon Gate Valve	Red	Syringe used to inflate balloon for placement and obtaining wedge values
Thermistor Connector	White/ Red	Measures blood temperature 4 cm from distal tip

Additional Swan-Ganz Catheters

LOCATION	COLOR	FUNCTION
Venous Infusion Port (VIP)	White	Additional RA lumen for fluid infusion
Venous Infusion Port (VIP+)	Purple	Additional RV lumen for fluid infusion
RV Pacing Lumen (Paceport)	Orange	Additional lumen for RV pacing or fluid infusion
RA Pacing Lumen (AV Paceport)	Yellow	Additional lumen for RA pacing or infusion of fluids

Port exit locations may vary depending on catheter model. See Swan-Ganz Catheter Reference Section.

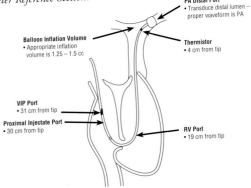

PA Distal Port
• Transduce distal lumen – proper waveform is PA

Balloon Inflation Volume
• Appropriate inflation volume is 1.25 – 1.5 cc

Thermistor
• 4 cm from tip

VIP Port
• 31 cm from tip

Proximal Injectate Port
• 30 cm from tip

RV Port
• 19 cm from tip

Normal Insertion Pressures and Waveform Tracings

Right Atrial/Central Venous Pressure (RA/CVP)

-1 to +7 mmHg

Mean 4 mmHg

a = atrial systole
c = backward bulging from tricuspid valve closure
v = atrial filling, ventricular systole

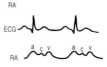

Right Ventricular

Systolic Pressure (RVSP)
15 - 25 mmHg
Diastolic Pressure (RVDP)
0 - 8 mmHg

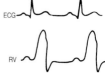

Pulmonary Artery

Systolic Pressure (PASP)
15 - 25 mmHg
Diastolic Pressure (PADP)
8 - 15 mmHg
Mean Pressure (MPA)
10 - 20 mmHg

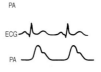

Pulmonary Artery Wedge Pressure (PAWP)

Mean 6 - 12 mmHg

a = atrial systole
v = atrial filling, ventricular systole

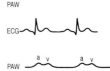

Abnormal Waveform Chart

RIGHT ATRIAL WAVEFORMS

Decreased mean pressure
Hypovolemia
Transducer zero level too high

Elevated mean pressure
Fluid overload states
Right ventricular failure
Left ventricular failure causing right ventricular failure
Tricuspid stenosis or regurgitation
Pulmonic stenosis or regurgitation
Pulmonary hypertension

Elevated "a" wave: atrial systole, increased resistance to ventricular filling
Tricuspid stenosis
Decreased right ventricular compliance
Right ventricular failure
Pulmonic stenosis
Pulmonary hypertension

Absent "a" wave
Atrial fibrillation
Atrial flutter
Junctional rhythms: cannon "a" waves

Elevated "v" wave: atrial filling, regurgitant flow
Tricuspid regurgitation
Functional regurgitation from right ventricular failure

Elevated "a" and "v" waves
Cardiac tamponade
Constrictive pericardial disease
Hypervolemia
Right ventricular failure

Abnormal Waveform Chart (continued)

RIGHT VENTRICULAR WAVEFORMS

Elevated systolic pressure
Pulmonary hypertension
Pulmonic valve stenosis
Factors that increase pulmonary vascular resistance

Decreased systolic pressure
Hypovolemia
Cardiogenic shock
Cardiac tamponade

Increased diastolic pressure
Hypervolemia
Congestive heart failure
Cardiac tamponade
Pericardial constriction

Decreased diastolic pressure
Hypovolemia

PULMONARY ARTERY WAVEFORMS

Elevated systolic pressure
Pulmonary disease
Increased pulmonary vascular resistance
Mitral stenosis or regurgitation
Left heart failure
Increased blood flow; left to right shunt

Reduced systolic pressure
Hypovolemia
Pulmonic stenosis
Tricuspid stenosis

Abnormal Waveform Chart (continued)

PULMONARY ARTERY WEDGE/LEFT ATRIAL WAVEFORM

Decreased mean pressure

Hypovolemia
Transducer zero level too high

Elevated mean pressure

Fluid overload states
Left ventricular failure
Mitral stenosis or regurgitation
Aortic stenosis or regurgitation
Myocardial infarction

Elevated "a" wave (any increased resistance to ventricular filling)

Mitral stenosis

Absent "a" wave

Atrial fibrillation
Atrial flutter
Junctional rhythms: Cannon "a" waves

Elevated "v" wave

Mitral regurgitation
Functional regurgitation from left ventricular failure
Ventricular septal defect

Elevated "a" and "v" waves

Cardiac tamponade
Constrictive pericardial disease
Left ventricular failure
Volume overload

Insertion Techniques for the Swan-Ganz Catheter

1. Before insertion of the Swan-Ganz catheter, prepare the pressure monitoring system for use according to the institution's policies and procedures.

2. Insert the catheter following recommended guidelines and advance the catheter towards the thorax.

3. Once the catheter tip has exited the introducer sheath (approximately 15 cm) and reached the junction of the superior or inferior vena cava and right atrium, the balloon is inflated with air or CO_2 to the full volume indicated on the catheter shaft and gate valve is locked (7 to 7.5F; 1.5 cc). This position can be noted when respiratory oscillations are seen on the monitor screen.

4. Catheter advancement to the PA should be rapid, since prolonged manipulation can result in loss of catheter stiffness. The Swan-Ganz catheter is made of a patented polyvinyl chloride (PVC) material designed to soften in vivo. With prolonged insertion times, a "softer" catheter may cause coiling in the RV or difficulties in catheter advancement.

5. Once the wedge position has been identified, the balloon is deflated by unlocking the gate valve, removing the syringe and allowing the back pressure in the PA to deflate the balloon. After balloon deflation, reattach the syringe to the gate valve. The gate valve is typically only placed in the locked position during catheter insertion.

6. To reduce or remove any redundant length or loop in the right atrium or ventricle, slowly pull the catheter back 1 – 2 cm. Then reinflate the balloon to determine the minimum inflation volume necessary to obtain a wedge pressure tracing. The catheter tip should be in a position where the full or near-full inflation volume (1.25 cc to 1.5 cc for 7 to 8F catheters) produces a wedge pressure tracing.

Catheter Insertion Distance Markings*

LOCATION	DISTANCE TO VC/RA JUNCTION	DISTANCE TO PA
Internal Jugular	15 to 20	40 to 55
Subclavian Vein	10 to 15	35 to 50
Femoral Vein	30	60
Right Antecubital Fossa	40	70
Left Antecubital Fossa	50	80

*(in cm)

Note: Catheter markings occur every 10 cms and are denoted by a thin black line. 50 cm markings are denoted by a thick black line. Catheter must exit introducer sheath before inflating balloon, approximately 15 cm of catheter length.

Tracings noted on insertion. Observe diastolic pressure on insertion as pressures will rise when pulmonary artery reached.

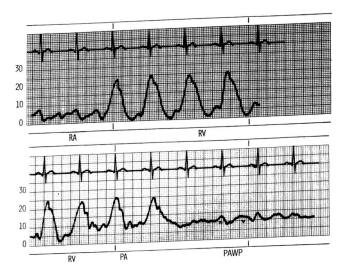

Continuous Pulmonary Artery Pressure Monitoring

1. Optimize pressure monitoring systems according to manufacturers' recommendations.
2. Maintain patency of inner lumens with heparinized solution or continuous flush systems.
3. Observe waveforms for proper placement.
4. Catheter migration may occur. Note any damping or loss of clarity of the PA tracing as catheter position may have changed.
5. Catheter may slip back to RV. Observe waveforms for spontaneous RV tracings from catheter slipping back into RV. Note changes in the diastolic pressure.
6. Wedge the catheter with the minimum balloon inflation volume required to obtain a wedge tracing. Note the inflation volume. If < 1.25 cc of volume is required, the catheter position may have changed. Consider repositioning the catheter.
7. Never use more than the recommended balloon inflation volume marked on the catheter shaft.
8. Never inflate the balloon more than the minimum required to obtain a wedge tracing.

*Catheter too distal
Overdamping of tracing.*

*Catheter spontaneous wedging
Wedge type tracing with
balloon deflated.*

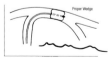

*Full inflation with 1.5 cc
inflation volume. Appropriate
"a" and "v" waves noted.*

*Overinflation of balloon.
Note waveform rise on screen.*

Physiological Rationale for Pulmonary Artery Pressure Monitoring

Ventricles in Systole

In this figure the balloon is deflated and the ventricles are in systole. The tricuspid and mitral valves are closed, while the pulmonic and aortic valves are open. A higher pressure is generated by the right ventricle during contraction and is transmitted to the catheter tip located in the pulmonary artery. The catheter records pulmonary artery systolic pressure (PASP), which reflects right ventricular systolic pressure (RVSP) because there is now a common chamber with a common volume and pressure.

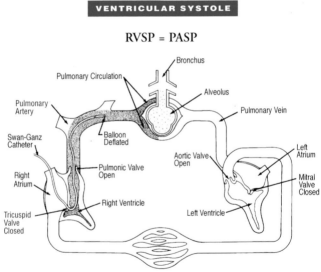

VENTRICULAR SYSTOLE

RVSP = PASP

Physiological Rationale for Pulmonary Artery Pressure Monitoring (continued)

Ventricles in diastole

During diastole the tricuspid and mitral valves are open. The ventricles are filling with blood from their respective atria. At this time the tricuspid valve (TV) and mitral valve (MV) are open and the pulmonic valve (PV) and aortic valve (AoV) are closed.

With the balloon still deflated, pulmonary artery diastolic pressure (PADP) is recorded. After the closure of the pulmonic valve, the right ventricle continues to relax. This causes a lower diastolic pressure in the right ventricle than in the pulmonary artery. RVEDP is less than PADP.

Since there is normally no obstruction between the pulmonary artery and left atrium, the pressure recorded will be virtually the same as left atrial pressure. Left atrial pressure is also reflected as left ventricular end-diastolic pressure (LVEDP) when the mitral valve is open.

When transducing the proximal port, the right atrial pressure reflects right ventricular end-diastolic pressure when the tricuspid valve is open.

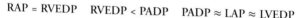

VENTRICULAR DIASTOLE

$$RAP = RVEDP \quad RVEDP < PADP \quad PADP \approx LAP \approx LVEDP$$

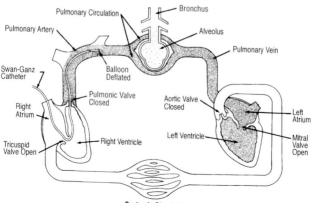

Pulmonary Circulation — Bronchus

Pulmonary Artery

Alveolus

Pulmonary Vein

Swan-Ganz Catheter

Balloon Deflated

Aortic Valve Closed

Right Atrium

Pulmonic Valve Closed

Left Atrium

Tricuspid Valve Open

Right Ventricle

Left Ventricle

Mitral Valve Open

Systemic Circulation

Physiological Rationale for Pulmonary Artery Pressure Monitoring

VENTRICLES IN DIASTOLE: CATHETER WEDGED

By inflating the balloon, the catheter floats downstream into a smaller branch of the pulmonary artery. Once the balloon lodges, the catheter is considered "wedged". It is in this wedge position that right sided and PA diastolic pressures are effectively occluded.

Because there are no valves between the pulmonic and mitral valve, there is now an unrestricted vascular channel between the catheter tip in the pulmonary artery through the pulmonary vascular bed, the pulmonary vein, the left atrium, the open mitral valve and into the left ventricle. The distal lumen is now more closely monitoring left ventricular filling pressure or left ventricular end-diastolic pressure.

The importance of this pressure is that normally it closely approximates the pressure present in the left ventricle during end-diastole and provides an indirect means of assessing left ventricular preload.

VENTRICULAR DIASTOLE

PAWP ≈ LAP ≈ LVEDP

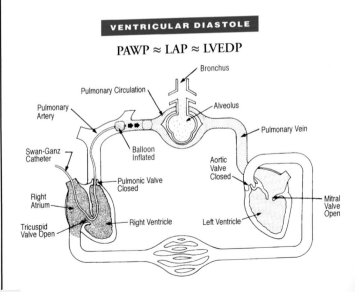

Normal Pressures and Oxygen Saturation Values

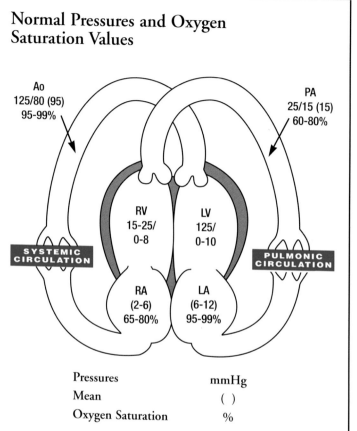

Ao
125/80 (95)
95-99%

PA
25/15 (15)
60-80%

RV
15-25/
0-8

LV
125/
0-10

SYSTEMIC
CIRCULATION

PULMONIC
CIRCULATION

RA
(2-6)
65-80%

LA
(6-12)
95-99%

Pressures	mmHg
Mean	( )
Oxygen Saturation	%

See "Normals Section" for full listing of Normal Ranges.

Cardiac Output Definition

Cardiac output (liters/minute, L/min): amount of blood ejected from the ventricle in a minute.

Cardiac Output = Heart Rate x Stroke Volume

Heart Rate = beats/min

Stroke Volume = ml/beat; amount of blood ejected from ventricle in one beat

CO = HR x SV ÷ 1000

Normal Cardiac Output: 4 - 8 L/min

Normal Cardiac Index : 2.5 - 4 L/min/M2

CI = CO/BSA

BSA = Body Surface Area

Normal Heart Rate Range: 60-100 BPM

Normal Stroke Volume: 60-100 ml

Stroke volume: difference between end-diastolic volume (EDV), [the amount of blood in the ventricle at the end of diastole], and end-systolic volume (ESV), [blood volume in the ventricle at the end of systole]. Normal SV is 60 to 100 ml/beat.

SV = EDV- ESV   SV also calculated by: **SV = CO/HR x 1000**

When stroke volume is expressed as a percentage of end-diastolic volume, stroke volume is referred to as the ejection fraction (EF). Normal ejection fraction for the LV is 60 - 75%. The normal EF for the RV is 40 - 60%. **EF = SV / EDV x 100**

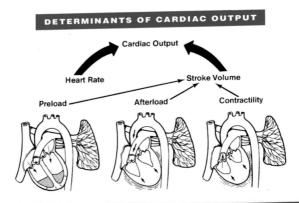

DETERMINANTS OF CARDIAC OUTPUT

Cardiac Output

Heart Rate → Stroke Volume

Preload   Afterload   Contractility

Preload Definition and Measurements

Preload refers to the amount of myocardial fiber stretch at the end of diastole. Preload also refers to the amount of volume in the ventricle at the end of this phase. It has been clinically acceptable to measure the pressure required to fill the ventricles as an indirect assessment of ventricular preload. Left atrial filling pressure (LAFP) or pulmonary artery wedge pressure (PAWP) and left atrial pressures (LAP) have been used to evaluate left ventricular preload. Right atrial pressure (RAP) have been used to assess right ventricular preload. Volumetric parameters (RVEDV) provide a closer measurement to ventricular preload for the right ventricle.

PRELOAD

RAP/CVP:	2 - 6 mm Hg
PAD:	8 - 15 mm Hg
PAWP/LAP:	6 - 12 mm Hg
RVEDV:	100 - 160 ml

Frank-Starling Law

Frank and Starling (1895, 1914) identified the relationship between myocardial fiber length and force of contraction. The more the diastolic volume or fiber stretch at the end of the diastole, the stronger the next contraction during systole to a physiologic limit.

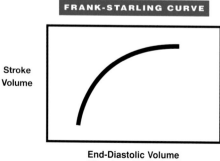

FRANK-STARLING CURVE

Stroke Volume

End-Diastolic Volume
Fiber Length, Preload

Ventricular Compliance Curves

The relationship between end-diastolic volume and end-diastolic pressure is dependent upon the compliance of the muscle wall. The relationship between the two is curvilinear. With normal compliance, relatively large increases in volume create relatively small increases in pressure. This will occur in a ventricle that is not fully dilated. When the ventricle becomes more fully dilated, smaller increases in volume produce greater rises in pressure. In a non-compliant ventricle, a greater pressure is generated with very little increase in volume. Increased compliance of the ventricle allows for large changes in volume with little rise in pressure.

EFFECTS OF VENTRICULAR COMPLIANCE

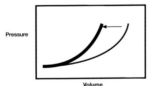

Normal Compliance
Pressure/volume relationship is curvilinear:

a: Large increase in volume = small increase in pressure

b: Small increase in volume = large increase in pressure

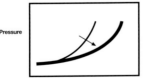

Decreased Compliance
Stiffer, less elastic ventricle
Ischemia
Increased afterload
Inotropes
Restrictive cardiomyopathies
Increased intrathoracic pressure
Increased pericardial pressure
Increased abdominal pressure

Increased Compliance
Less stiff, more elastic ventricle
Dilated cardiomyopathies
Decreased afterload
Vasodilators

Afterload Definition and Measurements

Afterload refers to the tension developed by the myocardial muscle fibers during ventricular systolic ejection. More commonly, afterload is described as the resistance, impedance, or pressure that the ventricle must overcome to eject its blood volume. Afterload is determined by a number of factors, including: volume and mass of blood ejected, the size and wall thickness of the ventricle, and the impedance of the vasculature. In the clinical setting, the most sensitive measure of afterload is systemic vascular resistance (SVR) for the left ventricle and pulmonary vascular resistance (PVR) for the right ventricle. The formulae for calculating afterload include the gradient difference between the beginning or inflow of the circuit and the end or outflow of the circuit.

AFTERLOAD

Pulmonary Vascular Resistance (PVR): <250 dynes/sec/cm-5

$$PVR = \frac{MPAP-PAWP}{CO} \times 80$$

Systemic Vascular Resistance (SVR): 800-1200 dynes/sec/cm-5

$$SVR = \frac{MAP-RAP}{CO} \times 80$$

Afterload has an inverse relationship to ventricular function. As resistance to ejection increases, the force of contraction decreases, resulting in a decreased stroke volume. As resistance to ejection increases, an increase in myocardial oxygen consumption occurs.

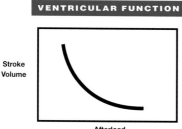

VENTRICULAR FUNCTION

Stroke Volume

Afterload

Contractility Definition and Measurements

Inotropism or contractility refers to the inherent property of the myocardial muscle fibers to shorten without altering the fiber length or preload.

Contractility changes can be plotted on a curve. It is important to note that changes in contractility result in shifts of the curves, but not the underlying basic shape.

Measurements of contractility can not be directly obtained. Clinical assessment parameters are surrogates and all include determinants of preload and afterload.

CONTRACTILITY

Stroke Volume	60-100 ml/beat
$SV = (CO \times 1000)/HR$	
$SVI = SV/BSA$	33-47 ml/beat/m2
Left Ventricular Stroke Work Index	50-62 gms-m/beat/m2
$LVSWI = SVI \ (MAP-PAWP) \times 0.0136$	
Right Ventricular Stroke Work Index	5-10 gms-m/m2/beat
$RVSWI = SVI \ (MPAP-RAP) \times 0.0136$	
Left Cardiac Work	3.8 ± 0.4 kg-m/m2
$LCW = CI \times MAP \times 0.0144$	
Right Cardiac Work	0.6 ± 0.6 kg-m/m2
$RCW = CI \times MPAP \times 0.0144$	

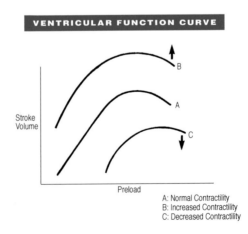

VENTRICULAR FUNCTION CURVE

A: Normal Contractility
B: Increased Contractility
C: Decreased Contractility

Family of Ventricular Function Curves

Ventricular function can be represented by a family of curves. The performance characteristics of the heart can move from one curve to another, depending upon the state of preload, afterload, contractility or ventricular compliance.

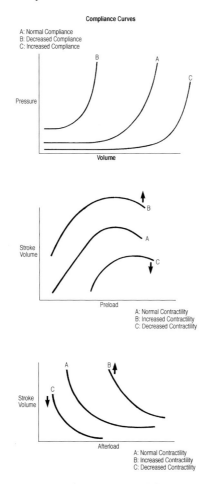

Compliance Curves

A: Normal Compliance
B: Decreased Compliance
C: Increased Compliance

Pressure

Volume

Stroke Volume

Preload

A: Normal Contractility
B: Increased Contractility
C: Decreased Contractility

Stroke Volume

Afterload

A: Normal Contractility
B: Increased Contractility
C: Decreased Contractility

Cardiac Output Determinations

There are three common indirect methods for cardiac output determinations: Fick, dye indicator dilution, and the thermodilution indicator method. The first two are primarily performed in a controlled catheterization laboratory setting. Thermodilution is most readily used at the bedside.

The Fick Method

The "gold standard" for cardiac output determinations is based on the principles developed by Adolph Fick in the 1870's. Fick's concept proposes that the uptake or release of a substance by an organ is the product of blood flow through that organ and the difference between the arterial and venous values of the same substance.

The Fick method utilizes oxygen as the substance and the lungs as the organ. Arterial and venous oxygen content are measured to obtain the difference (a - v O_2). Oxygen consumption (VO_2) can be calculated from the inspired minus expired oxygen content and ventilation rate. The cardiac output can then be determined using this formula:

$$\text{Cardiac Output} = \frac{\text{Oxygen Consumption in ml/min}}{\text{a - v } O_2 \text{ Difference in vol\%}}$$

(volume % = 1 ml oxygen/100 cc)

- Normal (CaO_2) arterial oxygen content: 20 volume %
- Normal (CvO_2) mixed venous oxygen content: 15 volume %
- Normal (VO_2) oxygen consumption: 250 ml/min

Inserting these values into the equation:
CO = 250 / (20 - 5) x 100
    = 250 / 5 x 100
    = 5000 ml/min or 5 l/min

Calculating cardiac output with the Fick equation requires accurate measurement of the oxygenation variables. Slight errors in the content values may produce large errors in the oxygen consumption result. Normal oxygen consumption ranges between 200 - 250 ml/min. Indexed normal VO_2 values are 110 - 130 ml/min/m2. Critically ill patients may not have normal oxygen consumption values; therefore, insertion of normal values into the above Fick equation may produce erroneous cardiac output values.

Dye Indicator Dilution Method

Principles for the indicator dilution method were first proposed in the 1890's by Stewart, and later refined by Hamilton.

The basis of the dye indicator technique is that a known concentration of an indicator is added to a body of fluid. After allowing adequate mixing time, the dilution of that indicator will produce the amount of fluid it was added to. A densimeter records the dye or indicator concentration in the blood after a known sample was injected upstream.

By taking continuous blood samples, a time-concentration plot, called an indicator-dilution curve can be obtained. Once this is plotted, the cardiac output can be calculated using the Stewart-Hamilton Equation:

$$CO = \frac{I \times 60}{Cm \times t} \times \frac{1}{k}$$

WHERE:

CO = cardiac output (l/min)
I = amount of dye injected (mg)
60 = 60 sec/min
Cm = mean indicator concentration (mg/l)
t = total curve duration (sec)
k = calibration factor (mg/ml/mm deflection)

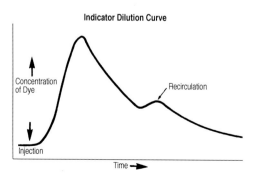

Indicator Dilution Curve

Thermodilution Method

In the early 1970's, Drs. Swan and Ganz demonstrated reliability and reproducibility of the thermodilution method with a special temperature sensing pulmonary artery catheter. Since that time, the thermodilution method of obtaining cardiac output has become a gold standard for clinical practice.

The thermodilution method applies indicator dilution principles, using temperature change as the indicator. A known amount of solution with a known temperature is injected rapidly into the proximal injectate lumen of the catheter. This cooler than blood temperature solution mixes with the surrounding blood, and the temperature is measured downstream in the pulmonary artery by a thermistor bead embedded in the catheter. The resultant change in temperature is then plotted on a time-temperature curve. This curve is similar to the one produced by the indicator-dilution method.

A modified Stewart-Hamilton equation is used to calculate the cardiac output taking into consideration the change in temperature as the indicator. Modifications include the measured temperature of the injectate and the patient's blood temperature, along with the specific gravity of the solution injected.

$$CO = \frac{V \times (TB - TI)}{A} \times \frac{(SI \times CI)}{(SB \times CB)} \times \frac{60 \times CT \times K}{1}$$

WHERE:

CO	= cardiac output
V	= volume of injectate (ml)
A	= area of thermodilution curve in square mm divided by paper speed (mm/sec)
K	= calibration constant in mm/°C
TB, TI	= temperature of blood (B) and injectate (I)
SB, SI	= specific gravity of blood and injectate
CB, CI	= specific heat of blood and injectate
$\frac{(SI \times CI)}{(SB \times CB)}$	= 1.08 when 5% dextrose is used
60	= 60 sec/min
CT	= correction factor for injectate warming

Thermodilution Curves

A normal curve characteristically shows a sharp upstroke from rapid injection of the injectate. This is followed by a smooth curve and slightly prolonged downslope back to the baseline. Since this curve represents a change from warmer temperature to cooler and then back to warmer temperature, the actual curve is in a negative direction. The area under the curve is inversely proportional to the cardiac output.

When cardiac output is low, more time is required for the temperature to return to baseline, producing a larger area under the curve. With high cardiac output, the cooler injectate is carried more quickly through the heart, and the temperature returns to baseline faster. This produces a smaller area under the curve.

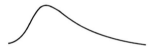

Normal Cardiac Output

Artifact Due to Noise Interference

High Cardiac Output

Low Cardiac Output

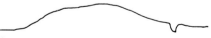

Improper Injection Technique

Troubleshooting Key Factors in Optimizing Bolus CO Determinations

The chart below describes factors that can influence the accuracy and reproducibility of bolus thermodilution cardiac output values.

	FACTOR AFFECTING ACCURACY OF BOLUS CO MEASUREMENT	POTENTIAL ERROR
	Inaccurate Injectate Temperature:	
	• 1°C error in iced injectate	± 2.7%
	• 1°C error in room temperature injectate	± 7.7%
	If injectate is removed from the ice bath for:	
	• 15 seconds	mean increase of 0.34 ± 0.16°C
	• 30 seconds	mean increase of 0.56 ± 0.18°C
	Inaccurate Injectate Volume	0.5 ml of error in 5 ml injection: ±10%
		0.5 ml of error in 10 ml injection: ± 5%
	Rapid Volume Infusion During Bolus Injections:	
	• Room temperature infusion	CO decreased 30-80%
	• Warmed infusion	CO decreased 20-40%
	Respiratory Cycle Influences	normal variance from 29-58% maximum variance up to 70%
	Inaccurate Computation Constant	1-100%
	Thermal Instability Post Cardiopulmonary Bypass(CPB):	
	• 1-10 minutes post	10-20%
	• 30 minutes post	up to 9%

Thermodilution Continuous Cardiac Output

By adapting intermittent thermodilution principles, continuous cardiac output (CCO) can now be obtained at the bedside. The system consists of a modified Swan-Ganz catheter and a sophisticated cardiac output computer.

The catheter has a special 10 cm length thermal filament which lies between the RA and RV when the catheter is correctly positioned. The energy signal is emitted from this thermal filament. The proximal injectate port is located 26 cm from the distal tip for observation of RA tracings.

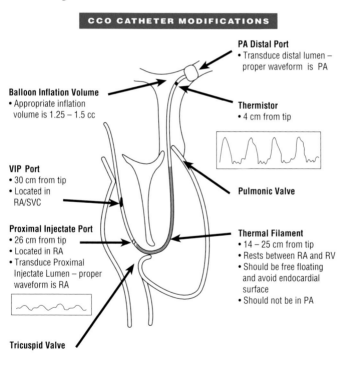

CCO CATHETER MODIFICATIONS

PA Distal Port
• Transduce distal lumen – proper waveform is PA

Balloon Inflation Volume
• Appropriate inflation volume is 1.25 – 1.5 cc

Thermistor
• 4 cm from tip

VIP Port
• 30 cm from tip
• Located in RA/SVC

Pulmonic Valve

Proximal Injectate Port
• 26 cm from tip
• Located in RA
• Transduce Proximal Injectate Lumen – proper waveform is RA

Thermal Filament
• 14 – 25 cm from tip
• Rests between RA and RV
• Should be free floating and avoid endocardial surface
• Should not be in PA

Tricuspid Valve

Continuous Cardiac Output Thermodilution Algorithm

Rather than using an injectate that is cooler than blood temperature for the input signal, as is done with the intermittent method, the catheter has a 10 cm thermal filament that emits pulses of energy in a repetitive on-off sequence. The sophisticated computer algorithm identifies when the pulmonary artery temperature change matches the input signal. Cross correlation of the input and output signal produces a thermodilution wash-out curve. The modified Stewart-Hamilton equation is applied to determine the cardiac output value. This process occurs approximately every 30-60 seconds and the values are averaged to produce a continuously displayed parameter. By using CCO technology many of the sources of error associated with the bolus technique are eliminated.

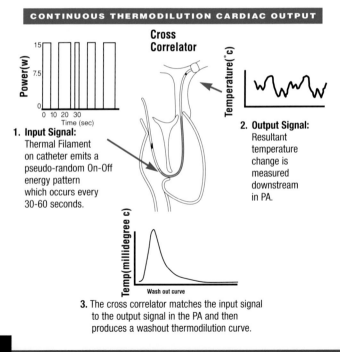

CONTINUOUS THERMODILUTION CARDIAC OUTPUT

Cross Correlator

1. **Input Signal:**
   Thermal Filament on catheter emits a pseudo-random On-Off energy pattern which occurs every 30-60 seconds.

2. **Output Signal:**
   Resultant temperature change is measured downstream in PA.

Wash out curve

3. The cross correlator matches the input signal to the output signal in the PA and then produces a washout thermodilution curve.

Vigilance Monitor

The Vigilance monitor can be used to view the trended cardiac output values over time. With the addition of SvO₂, dual trends can be observed.

HOME SCREEN

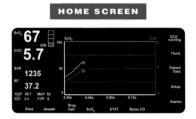

Analog inputs of MAP and CVP can provide the clinician with on-line continuous SVR or SVRI values. When analog SaO₂ is available, dual oximetry values, such as O_2EI or VQI can be displayed.

ANESTHESIA SCREEN

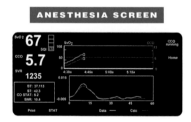

The STAT Mode Screen provides the clinician with a more rapid assessment of the cardiac output values obtained. This screen is frequently used when therapeutic changes are being assessed.

STAT MODE SCREEN

Right Ventricular Volumetrics and Ejection Fraction

Right ventricular volumetric and ejection fraction (EF) assessment utilizes technology similar to standard thermodilution techniques. Modifications include a fast response thermistor, which potentiates sensing of changes in PA temperatures. A multihole injectate lumen is present in the main body of the right atrium to facilitate homogeneous mixing of blood and injectate. The modified computer requires the input of the heart rate, either sensed by intra-cardiac electrodes or slaved in from the bedside ECG.

The methodology of EF calculation is similar to that of thermodilution CO. Whereas CO is dependent upon the change in temperature sensed over time, EF is dependent upon a beat-to-beat change in temperature. To determine RV EF, the thermistor senses changes of temperature and gates the change in temperature with an R wave. By assessing the change of temperature at two different beats as well as the number of beats occurring in the interval between the two temperatures, the computer is able to calculate EF, or the percent of blood ejected with each beat. Once EF is obtained, the computer determines the SV (SV = CO/HR x 1000) and calculates EDV (EDV = SV/EF).

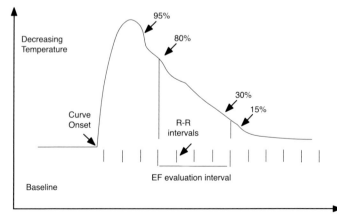

Normal RV Volumetric Parameters

Right Ventricular Ejection Fraction
Normal RV EF   40 - 60%

Right Ventricular End-Diastolic Volume (EDV = SV/EF)
Normal RV EDV   100 - 160 ml
Normal RV EDVI   60 - 100 ml/m2

Right Ventricular End-Systolic Volume (ESV = EDV - SV)
Normal RV ESV   50 - 100 ml
Normal RV ESVI   30 - 60 ml/m2

Stroke Volume (SV = CO/HR x 1000)
Normal SV   60 - 100 ml
Normal SVI   35 - 60 ml/m2

Pulmonary Function Tests

DEFINITIONS

Total Lung Capacity (TLC): maximal amount of air within the lung at maximal inspiration. (6.0L)

Vital Capacity (VC): maximal amount of air that can be exhaled after a maximal inspiration. (4.5L)

Forced Vital Capacity (FVC): maximal amount of air exhaled after previous maximal expiratory effort. (1.5L)

Inspiratory Capacity (IC): maximal amount of air that can be inhaled from resting level after normal expiration. (3.0L)

Inspiratory Reserve Volume (IRV): maximal amount of air that can be inhaled after a normal inspiration during quiet breathing. (2.5L)

Expiratory Reserve Volume (ERV): maximal amount of air that can be exhaled from the resting level following a normal expiration. (1.5L)

Functional Residual Capacity (FRC): amount of air remaining in the lungs at the end of normal expiration. (3.0L)

Residual Volume (RV): volume of gas remaining in lungs after maximal expiration. (1.5L)

NORMAL SPIROGRAM

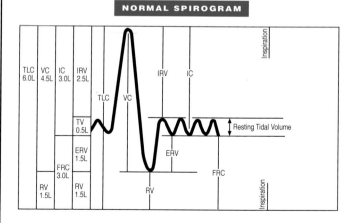

Acid Base Balance

Simple acid base abnormalities can be divided into metabolic and respiratory disorders. Values obtained from blood gas analysis can assist in determining the disorder present.

DEFINITIONS:

Acid: A substance which can donate hydrogen ions
Base: A substance which can accept hydrogen ions.
pH: The "power of hydrogen".
Acidemia: An acid condition of the blood with pH < 7.35
Alkalemia: An alkaline (base) condition of the blood with pH > 7.45

PCO_2: Respiratory Component
$PaCO_2$: Normal ventilation 35 - 45 mm Hg
      Hypoventilation > 45 mm Hg
      Hyperventilation < 35 mm Hg

HCO_3: Metabolic Component
      Balanced 22 - 26 mEq/L
        Base Balance - 2 to +2
        Metabolic Alkalosis > 26 mEq/L
          Base excess > +2 mEq/L
        Metabolic Acidosis < 22 mEq/L
          Base deficit < 2 mEq/L

NORMAL BLOOD GAS VALUES

Component	Arterial	Venous
pH	7.40 (7.35 - 7.45)	7.36 (7.31 - 7.41)
PO_2 mmHg	80 - 100	35 - 45
SO_2%	95 or >	60 - 80
PCO_2 mmHg	35 - 45	41 - 51
HCO_3 mEq/L	22 - 26	22 - 26
Base excess/deficit	-2 - +2	-2 - +2

Oxyhemoglobin Dissociation Curve

The oxyhemoglobin dissociation curve (ODC) graphically illustrates the relationship that exists between the partial pressure (PO_2) of oxygen and oxygen saturation (SO_2). The sigmoid shaped curve can be divided into two segments. The association segment or upper portion of the curve represents oxygen uptake in the lungs or the arterial side. The dissociation segment is the lower portion of the curve and represents the venous side, where oxygen is released from the hemoglobin.

NORMAL OXYHEMOGLOBIN DISSOCIATION CURVE

The affinity of hemoglobin for oxygen is independent of the PO_2-SO_2 relationship. Under normal conditions, the point at which the hemoglobin is 50% saturated with oxygen is called the P50 at a PO_2 of 27 mmHg. Alterations in the hemoglobin-oxygen affinity will produce shifts in the ODC.

FACTORS SHIFTING OXYHEMOGLOBIN DISSOCIATION CURVE

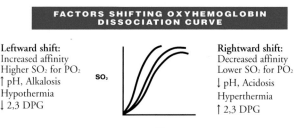

Leftward shift:
Increased affinity
Higher SO_2 for PO_2
↑ pH, Alkalosis
Hypothermia
↓ 2,3 DPG

Rightward shift:
Decreased affinity
Lower SO_2 for PO_2
↓ pH, Acidosis
Hyperthermia
↑ 2,3 DPG

The clinical significance of shifting the ODC is that SO_2 and PO_2 assessment parameters may not accurately reflect the patients' clinical status. A shift of the ODC to the left can lead to tissue hypoxia in spite of normal or high saturation values.

Pulmonary Gas Exchange Equations

Assessing pulmonary function is an important step in determining the cardiorespiratory status of the critically ill patient. Certain equations can be employed to evaluate pulmonary gas exchange, to evaluate the diffusion of oxygen across the pulmonary capillary unit, and to determine the amount of intrapulmonary shunting. An alteration in any of these will impact oxygen delivery.

Alveolar Gas Equation: PAO_2 is known as the ideal alveolar PO_2 and is calculated knowing the composition of inspired air.

$$PAO_2 = (PB - PH_2O) \times FiO_2 - PaCO_2 \times [FiO_2 + (1- FiO_2)/0.8]$$

Alveolar-arterial Oxygen Gradient: (A-a Gradient or P(A-a) O_2)

$P(A-a)O_2$: Assesses the amount of oxygen diffusion across the alveolar capillary unit. Compares the alveolar gas equation to the arterial partial pressure of oxygen.

$$[(PB - PH_2O) \times FiO_2] - PaCO_2 \times [FiO_2 + (1- FiO_2)/0.8] - (PaO_2)]$$

    Normal: < 15 mmHg on room air
    Normal : 60 - 70 mmHg on FiO_2 1.0

PB: Atmospheric Pressure: 760
PH_2O: Pressure of water: 47 mm Hg
FiO_2: Fraction of inspired air
$PaCO_2$: Partial Pressure of CO_2
0.8: Respiratory Quotient

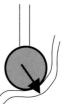

A-a GRADIENT CALCULATION

(Barometric Pressure	−	Water Vapor Pressure)	x	Patient's FiO_2	−	$\frac{PaCO_2}{0.8}$	−	Patient's PaO_2	
(760	−	47)	x	0.21	−	$\frac{40}{0.8}$	−	90	
	713		x	0.21	−	50	−	90	
				99.73			−	90	= 9.73
				A-a Gradient			≅	10	

Assumes breathing at sea level, on room air, with a $PaCO_2$ of 40 mm Hg and PaO_2 of 90 mm Hg.

Intrapulmonary Shunt

Intrapulmonary shunt (Qs/Qt) is defined as the amount of venous blood that by-passes an alveolar capillary unit and does not participate in oxygen exchange. Normally a small percentage of the blood flow drains directly into either the thebesian or pleural veins which exit directly into the left side of the heart. This is considered an anatomical or true shunt, and is approximately 1 – 2% in normal subjects and up to 5% in ill patients.

The physiologic shunt or capillary shunt occurs when there is either collapsed alveolar units or other conditions where the venous blood is not oxygenated.

Some controversies exist in regards to measuring Qs/Qt. A true shunt is said to be accurately measured only when the patient is on an FiO_2 of 1.0. Venous admixture which produces a physiologic shunt can be determined when the patient is on an FiO_2 of < 1.0. Both determinations require pulmonary artery saturation values to complete the calculation.

$$Qs/Qt = \frac{CcO_2 - CaO_2}{CcO_2 - CvO_2}$$

CcO_2 = Capillary oxygen content
$\qquad$ $(1.38 \times Hgb \times 1) + (PAO_2 \times 0.0031)$
CaO_2 = Arterial oxygen content
$\qquad$ $(1.38 \times Hgb \times SaO_2) + (PaO_2 \times 0.0031)$
CvO_2 = Venous oxygen content
$\qquad$ $(1.38 \times Hgb \times SvO_2) + (PvO_2 \times 0.0031)$

QS/QT

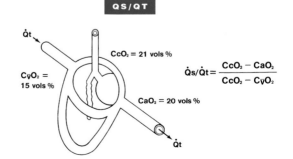

$\dot{Q}t$

$CcO_2 = 21$ vols %

$C\bar{v}O_2 = 15$ vols %

$\dot{Q}s/\dot{Q}t = \dfrac{CcO_2 - CaO_2}{CcO_2 - C\bar{v}O_2}$

$CaO_2 = 20$ vols %

$\dot{Q}t$

Intrapulmonary Shunt (continued)

Ventilation Perfusion Index (VQI) has been described as a dual oximetry estimate of intrapulmonary shunt (Qs/Qt). Assumptions involved in the equation are:

1. Dissolved oxygen is discounted
2. 100% saturation of pulmonary end-capillary blood
3. Hgb changes are not abrupt

Limitations of VQI include:
1. VQI can only be calculated if $SaO_2 < 100\%$
2. Poor agreement with Qs/Qt if $PaO_2 > 99$ mmHg
3. Good correlation when Qs/Qt > 15%

Equation Derivations:

$$Qs/Qt = \frac{100 \times [(1.38 \times Hgb) + (0.0031 \times PAO_2) - CaO_2)]}{[(1.38 \times Hgb) + (0.0031 \times PAO_2) - CvO_2)]}$$

$$VQI = \frac{100 \times [1.38 \times Hgb \times (1 - SaO_2/100) + (0.0031 \times PAO_2)}{[1.38 \times Hgb \times (1 - SvO_2/100) + (0.0031 \times PAO_2)}$$

Dual Oximetry: Simplifies the Shunt Equation

$$VQI = \frac{SAO_2 - SaO_2 = 1 - SaO_2 \text{ or } 1 - SpO_2}{SAO_2 - SvO_2 = 1 - SvO_2 \text{ or } 1 - SvO_2}$$

Oxygen Delivery
(DO_2 = CO_2 x CO x 10)

DO_2 is the amount of oxygen delivered or transported to the tissues in one minute and is comprised of oxygen content and the cardiac output. The adequacy of oxygen delivery is dependent upon appropriate pulmonary gas exchange, hemoglobin levels, sufficient oxygen saturation and cardiac output.

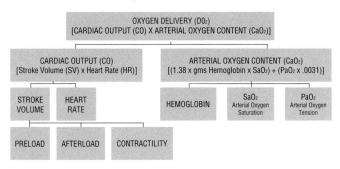

Oxygen Content (CO_2): amount of oxygen carried in the blood, both arterial and venous.

$$(1.38 \times Hgb \times SO_2) + (0.0031 \times PO_2)$$

1.38: amount of O_2 that can combine with 1 gram of hemoglobin
0.0031: solubility coefficient of O_2 in the plasma

$$CaO_2 = (1.38 \times Hgb \times SaO_2) + (0.0031 \times PaO_2)$$
Normal 20.1 ml/dl
$$CvO_2 = (1.38 \times Hgb \times SvO_2) + (0.0031 \times PvO_2)$$
Normal 5.5 ml/dl

Oxygen Delivery (DO_2): amount of oxygen transported in blood to tissues. Both arterial and venous O_2 delivery can be measured.

Arterial oxygen delivery (DaO_2): CO x CaO_2 x 10
$$5 \times 20.1 \times 10 = 1005 \text{ ml/min}$$
Venous oxygen delivery (DvO_2): CO x CvO_2 x 10
$$5 \times 15.5 \times 10 = 775 \text{ ml/min}$$

Oxygen Consumption

Oxygen consumption refers to the amount of oxygen used by the tissues; i.e., systemic gas exchange. This value cannot be measured directly but can be assessed by measuring the amount of oxygen delivered on the arterial side compared to the amount on the venous.

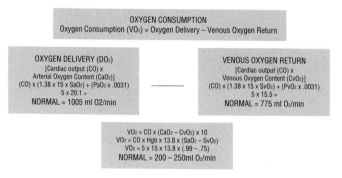

OXYGEN CONSUMPTION
Oxygen Consumption (VO$_2$) = Oxygen Delivery – Venous Oxygen Return

OXYGEN DELIVERY (DO$_2$)
[Cardiac output (CO) x
Arterial Oxygen Content (CaO$_2$)]
(CO) x (1.38 x 15 x SaO$_2$) + (PaO$_2$ x .0031)
5 x 20.1 =
NORMAL = 1005 ml O$_2$/min

VENOUS OXYGEN RETURN
[Cardiac output (CO) x
Venous Oxygen Content (CvO$_2$)]
(CO) x (1.38 x 15 x SvO$_2$) + (PvO$_2$ x .0031)
5 x 15.5 =
NORMAL = 775 ml O$_2$/min

VO$_2$ = CO x (CaO$_2$ – CvO$_2$) x 10
VO$_2$ = CO x Hgb x 13.8 x (SaO$_2$ – SvO$_2$)
VO$_2$ = 5 x 15 x 13.8 x (.99 – .75)
NORMAL = 200 – 250ml O$_2$/min

Oxygen Consumption: VO$_2$

Arterial Oxygen transport – Venous Oxygen Transport

$VO_2 = (CO \times CaO_2) - (CO \times CvO_2)$

$= CO (CaO_2 - CvO_2)$

$= CO [(SaO_2 \times Hgb \times 13.8) - (SvO_2 \times Hgb \times 13.8)]$

$= CO \times Hgb \times 13.8 \times (SaO_2 - SvO_2)$

Normals : 200 – 250 ml/min

100 – 125 ml/min/m2

Conditions and Activities Altering Demand and VO$_2$

Fever (one degree C)	10%	Work of Breathing	40%
Shivering	50-100%	Post Op Procedure	7%
ET Suctioning	7-70%	MSOF	20-80%
Sepsis	50-100%	Dressing Change	10%
Visitor	22%	Bath	23%
Position Change	31%	Chest X-Ray	25%
Sling Scale Weighing	36%		

Other Assessment Parameters for Oxygen Utilization

Arterial-Venous Oxygen Difference:
Ca-v O_2: normally 5 vol %
20 vol % - 15 vol % = 5 vol %

Oxygen Extraction Ratio:
O_2ER: normally 22 – 30 %
O_2ER: CaO_2 - CvO_2 / CaO_2 x 100
CaO_2 = 20.1 CvO_2 = 15.6
O_2ER = 20.1 - 15.6/20. 1 x 100 = 22.4%

Oxygen Extraction Index:
Dual oximetry estimate of oxygen extraction ratio. Evaluates the efficiency of oxygen extraction. Reflects cardiac reserve to increases in O_2 demand.
O_2EI = SaO_2 - SvO_2/SaO_2 x 100 (SaO_2 = 99, SvO_2 = 75)
O_2EI = 99 - 75/99 x 100 = 24.2%

CO vs SvO_2 Correlations
SvO_2 Reflects Balance Between Oxygen Delivery and Utilization Relationship to Fick Equation
VO_2 = C(a - v)O_2 x CO x 10
CO = VO_2/ C(a-v)O_2
C(a-v)O_2 = VO_2/CO
S(a-v)O_2 = VO_2/CO

When Fick equation is rearranged, the determinants of SvO_2 are the components of oxygen delivery and consumption:
If SaO_2 = 1.0 then SvO_2 = CvO_2/ CaO_2
SvO_2 = 1 - [VO_2/ (CO x 10 x CaO_2)]
SvO_2 = 1 - VO_2/ DO_2

As a result, SvO_2 reflects changes in oxygen extraction and the balance between DO_2 and VO_2.

VO₂/ DO₂ Relationships

The relationship between oxygen delivery and consumption can theoretically be plotted on a curve. Since normally the amount of oxygen delivered is approximately four times the amount consumed, the amount of oxygen required is independent of the amount delivered. This is the supply independent portion of the curve. If oxygen delivery decreases, the cells can extract more oxygen in order to maintain normal oxygen consumption levels. Once the compensatory mechanisms have been exhausted, the amount of oxygen consumed is now dependent on the amount delivered. This portion of the graph is called supply dependent.

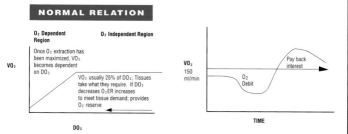

The concept of oxygen debt has gained more acceptance over the last decade. Oxygen debt occurs when the delivery of oxygen is insufficient to meet the body requirements. The implication of this concept is that additional oxygen delivery must be supported to "repay" this debt once it has occurred.

Factors Influencing Accumulation of O₂ Debt:

Oxygen Demand > Oxygen Consumed = Oxygen Debt
Decreased oxygen delivery
Decreased cellular oxygen extraction
Increased oxygen demands

Continuous Mixed Venous Oxygen Saturation Monitoring

REFLECTION SPECTROPHOTOMETRY

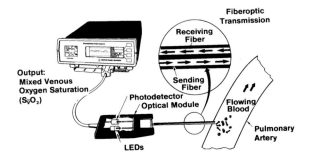

Output:
Mixed Venous
Oxygen Saturation
($S_{\bar{v}}O_2$)

Photodetector
Optical Module

LEDs

Fiberoptic
Transmission

Receiving
Fiber

Sending
Fiber

Flowing
Blood

Pulmonary
Artery

SWAN-GANZ OXIMETRY TD CATHETER

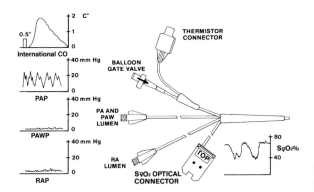

0.5°

International CO

2 C°
1
0

PAP

40 mm Hg
20
0

PAWP

40 mm Hg
20
0

RAP

40 mm Hg
20
0

THERMISTOR
CONNECTOR

BALLOON
GATE VALVE

PA AND
PAW
LUMEN

RA
LUMEN

$S_{\bar{v}}O_2$ OPTICAL
CONNECTOR

80
40

$S_{\bar{v}}O_2\%$

CCOmbo Monitoring Systems:
CCO and SvO₂ Continuous Display

VIGILANCE MONITOR

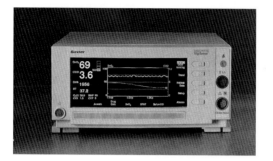

**PARAMETERS OBTAINED WITH
THE CCOmbo SYSTEM***

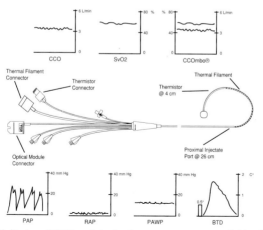

* Digital display of SVR and dual oximetry parameters available if
appropriate input variables provided.

Intra-arterial Monitoring

Components of Arterial Pulse

Peak Systolic Pressure: begins with opening of aortic valve. This reflects maximum left ventricular systolic pressure and may be termed the ascending limb.

Dicrotic Notch: closure of the aortic valve, marking the end of systole and the onset of diastole.

Diastolic Pressure: relates to the level of vessel recoil or amount of vasoconstriction in the arterial system. May be termed the descending limb.

Anacrotic Notch: A presystolic rise may be seen during the first phase of ventricular systole (isovolumetric contraction). The anacrotic notch will occur before the opening of the aortic valve.

Pulse Pressure: difference between systolic and diastolic pressure.

Mean Arterial Pressure: average pressure in the arterial system during a complete cardiac cycle. Systole requires one-third of the cardiac cycle, diastole normally during two-thirds. This timing relationship is reflected in the equation for calculating MAP. MAP = SP + (2DP)/3

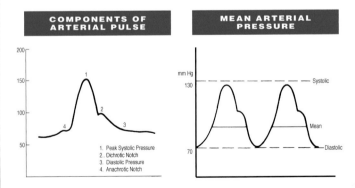

COMPONENTS OF ARTERIAL PULSE

1. Peak Systolic Pressure
2. Dicrotic Notch
3. Diastolic Pressure
4. Anacrotic Notch

MEAN ARTERIAL PRESSURE

mm Hg

130 — Systolic

— Mean

70 --- Diastolic

Intra-arterial Monitoring (continued)

ABNORMAL ARTERIAL PRESSURE WAVEFORMS

Elevated systolic pressure	Systemic hypertension
	Arteriosclerosis
	Aortic insufficiency
Decreased systolic pressure	Aortic stenosis
	Heart failure
	Hypovolemia
Widened pulse pressure	Systemic hypertension
	Aortic insufficiency
Narrowed pulse pressure	Cardiac tamponade
	Congestive heart failure
	Cardiogenic shock
	Aortic stenosis
Pulsus bisferiens	Aortic insufficiency
	Obstructive hypertrophic cardiomyopathy
Pulsus paradoxus	Cardiac tamponade
	Chronic obstructive airway disease
	Pulmonary embolism
Pulsus alternans	Congestive heart failure
	Cardiomyopathy

Pressure Monitoring Systems

This schematic identifies the components of a standard pressure monitoring system. The Swan-Ganz catheter and arterial catheter can be attached to a pressure monitoring line. The tubing must be non-compliant to accurately transmit the patient's pressure waves to the transducer. The disposable pressure transducer is kept patent by a pressurized solution (300 mmHg). An integral flush device with a restrictor limits the flow rate to approximately 3 cc/ hour for adults. Typically, heparinized normal saline is used as the flush solution with a range of heparin from 0.5u/1cc to 2u/1cc ratio. Non-heparinized solution has been used with patients with a sensitivity to heparin.

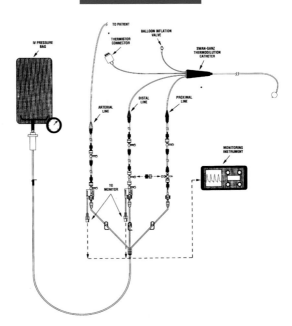

PRESSURE SYSTEM

IV PRESSURE BAG

TO PATIENT

THERMISTOR CONNECTOR

BALLOON INFLATION VALVE

SWAN-GANZ THERMODILUTION CATHETER

ARTERIAL LINE

DISTAL LINE

PROXIMAL LINE

MONITORING INSTRUMENT

TO MONITOR

Determining Dynamic Response

Optimal pressure monitoring requires a pressure system that accurately reproduces the physiologic signals applied to it. Dynamic response characteristics of the system includes the natural frequency and damping coefficient. Activate the flush device to perform a square wave test in order to measure the natural frequency and calculate the amplitude ratio.

Perform a Square Wave Test:

Activate the flush device by pulling the snap tab or pull tab. Observe the bedside monitor. The waveform will sharply rise and "square off" at the top. Observe the tracing as it returns to baseline.

Calculate the Natural Response (fn):

Estimated by measuring the time of one full oscillation (mm).

$$fn = \frac{\text{paper speed (mm/sec)}}{\text{oscillation width/ mm}}$$

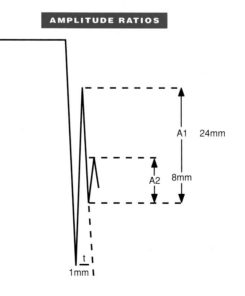

AMPLITUDE RATIOS

A1   24mm

A2   8mm

t

1mm

Determining Dynamic Response (continued)

Determine the Amplitude Ratio:

Estimate by measuring the amplitudes of two consecutive oscillations to determine an amplitude ratio, A2/ A1.

Plot to Determine Damping Coefficient:

Plot the natural frequency (fn) against the amplitude ratio to determine the damping coefficient. The amplitude ratio is on the right and the damping coefficient is on the left.

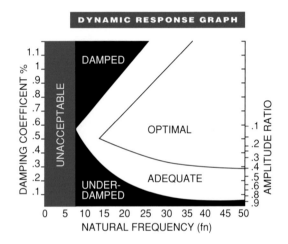

DYNAMIC RESPONSE GRAPH

Simple Evaluation of Dynamic Response

Determining the dynamic response characteristics of a pressure monitoring system by calculating the amplitude ratio and damping coefficient may not be feasible at the bedside when a rapid assessment of the waveform is required. A simple evaluation of dynamic response can be obtained by performing a square wave test and by observing the resultant oscillations. In order to perform this assessment accurately, a flush device that can be activated rapidly and then released is required. A flush device that does not close rapidly after activation (squeeze or press type) may not close the restrictor quickly and may produce erroneous results.

Square Wave Testing

1. Activate snap or pull tab on flush device.
2. Observe square wave generated on bedside monitor.
3. Count oscillations after square wave.
4. Observe distance between the oscillations.

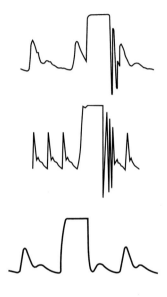

Optimally Damped:
1 - 2 oscillations before returning to tracing. Values obtained are accurate.

Underdamped:
> 2 oscillations. Overestimated systolic pressure, diastolic pressures may be underestimated.

Overdamped:
< 1 $1/2$ oscillations. Underestimation of systolic pressures, diastolic may not be affected.

Measuring Technique

Hydrostatic Zero Reference

To obtain accurate pressure measurements, the level of the air-fluid interface must be aligned with the chamber or vessel being measured.

The phlebostatic axis has been well defined as the appropriate landmark for intracardiac pressures. The phlebostatic axis has most recently been defined as the bisection of the 4th intercostal space at the mid-point between the anterior and posterior chest wall.

Physiologic pressures are measured relative to the atmospheric pressure. Therefore the transducer must be zeroed to the atmospheric pressure to eliminate its impact on the readings. Hydrostatic pressure occurs when the level of the zeroing stopcock is not in alignment with the phlebostatic axis.

The phlebostatic axis is used for both intracardiac and intra-arterial pressure monitoring. Accurate values can be obtained with the patient supine and with the head of bed up to 45 to 60 degrees as long as the zeroing stopcock has been aligned with the phlebostatic axis.

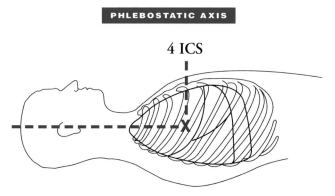

PHLEBOSTATIC AXIS

4 ICS

Mid-Point
A-P Chest Wall

Lung Zone Placement

Catheter tip location in relationship to lung zones may impact the validity of pulmonary artery wedge readings, both under normal conditions and with the application of PEEP. Lung zones are identified by the relationships among the inflow pressure (pulmonary artery pressure, PaP), the outflow pressure (pulmonary venous pressure, PvP), and the surrounding alveolar pressure (PAP).

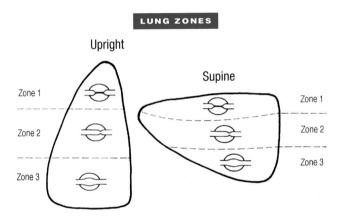

LUNG ZONES

Upright

Supine

Zone 1

Zone 2

Zone 3

Zone 1

Zone 2

Zone 3

Zone 1: PaP < PAP > PvP. No blood flow occurs from the collapsed pulmonary capillary beds. The Swan-Ganz catheter is a flow-directed catheter and the tip will not usually flow to this lung region. PAWP readings will be inaccurate.

Zone 2: PaP > PAP > PvP. Some blood flow occurs since the arterial pressure is greater than the alveolar pressure. Under some conditions catheter tip may reside in Zone 2 placement. PAWP readings may be inaccurate.

Zone 3: PaP > PAP < PvP. Capillaries are open resulting in blood flow. Catheter tip is usually below the level of the left atrium and can be verified by a lateral chest x-ray. PAWP readings will be accurate.

Lung Zone Placement (continued)

Guidelines for Optimal Lung Zone Catheter Placement

CRITERION	OPTIMAL ZONE 3	SUB-OPTIMAL ZONE 1 OR 2
Catheter tip location	Below level of LA	Above level of LA
Respiratory variations	Minimal	Marked
PAWP contour	"a" & "v" waves clearly present	"a" & "v" waves unclear
PAD versus PAWP	PAD > PAWP (normal physiology)	PAWP > PAD (no abnormal "a" & "v" waves present)
PEEP trial	Change in PAWP < $^1/_2$ change in PEEP	Change in PAWP > $^1/_2$ change in PEEP
Hydration status	Normovolemic	Hypovolemic

Ventilatory Effects on Pulmonary Artery Tracings

Spontaneous Breathing

During normal respiration, inspiration results in decreased intrathoracic pressure and increased venous return resulting in increased cardiac filling. However, the waveforms on inspiration will be negative due to the greater inspiratory decrease in intrathoracic pressure than the inspiratory increase in the cardiac volumes. On expiration, the intrathoracic pressure is relatively higher than on inspiration and will result in positive deflections in the PA and PAW waveforms. The values recorded should be obtained at end-expiration when the intrathoracic pressure influence is minimal.

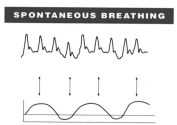

SPONTANEOUS BREATHING

Ventilatory Effects (continued)

Controlled Mechanical Ventilation

When a patient is ventilated and is not spontaneously breathing, the intrathoracic pressure during inspiration is at a positive level with ventilated breaths. On expiration, the values are negative due to the relative negative intrathoracic pressure at that phase. Again, the values, PA and PAW, are to be read at end-expiration.

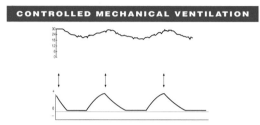

CONTROLLED MECHANICAL VENTILATION

Intermittent Mandatory Ventilation

When a form of intermittent mandatory ventilation is being applied, some breaths are controlled while others are spontaneous. The impact on the tracings is that during the controlled breaths, inspiration will produce elevated waves such as those during controlled mechanical ventilation. During a spontaneous breath the tracing will revert to normal with inspiration producing a negative wave. Observation of the patient's breathing and noting if the breaths are controlled or spontaneous assists in the proper identification of end-expiration values of pulmonary artery pressures.

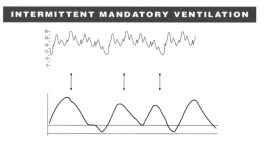

INTERMITTENT MANDATORY VENTILATION

Ventilatory Effects (continued)

This is a tracing of a patient who is spontaneously breathing. Identification of PA pressures and PAW pressures are influenced by the respiratory variations noted. Pressure values should be obtained at end-expiration. Possible causes for the respiratory variation includes hypovolemia or catheter tip in a non-zone 3 placement.

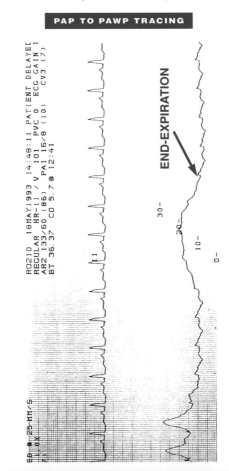

PAP TO PAWP TRACING

Concentrations in Frequently Used Intravenous Solutions (mEq/L)

FLUID	GLUCOSE	NA+	K+	CL-	MOSM/L	KCAL/L
D5W	50g	0	0	0	252	170
D10W	100g	0	0	0	505	340
D50W	500g	0	0	0	2520	1700
1/2 NS (0.45%NS)	0	77	0	77	154	0
NS (0.9% NS)	0	154	0	154	308	0
D51/4NS	50g	38	0	38	329	170
D5 1/2NS	50g	77	0	77	406	170
D5 NS	50g	154	0	154	560	170
LR	0	130	4	110	272	10

ATLS Chart

Estimated Fluid and Blood Requirements in a 70-kg Male

INITIAL PRESENTATIONS

	CLASS I	CLASS II	CLASS III	CLASS IV
Blood loss (mL)	<750	750-1500	1500-2000	≥2000
Blood loss (% blood volume)	<15	15-30	30-40	≥40
Pulse rate (bpm)	<100	>100	>120	≥140
Blood pressure	Normal	Normal	Decreased	Decreased
Pulse pressure (mm Hg)	Normal or increased	Decreased	Decreased	Decreased
Capillary blanch test	Normal	Positive	Positive	Positive
Respiratory rate	14-20	20-30	30-40	>35
Urine output (mL/hr)	30 or more	20-30	5-15	Negligible
CNS-mental status	Slightly anxious	Mildly anxious	Anxious and confused	Confused and lethargic
Fluid replacement	Crystalloid	Crystalloid	Crystalloid + blood	Crystalloid + blood

From Advanced Trauma Life Support Course, Instructor Manual. American College of Surgeons (ACS) Committee on Trauma, 1983/1984.

Fluid Challenge Guideline Chart

Baseline values:

PAWP* mmHg	CHALLENGE VOLUME AMOUNT/10 MINUTES	CVP* mmHg
< 12 mmHg	200 ml or 20 cc/minute	< 8 mmHg
12 - 16 - 18 mmHg	100 ml or 10 cc/minute	8 - 13 mmHg
> 16 - 18 mmHg	50 ml or 5 cc/ minute	> 13 mmHg

- Re-profile at the end of 10 minutes or fluid challenge.
- Discontinue challenge if PAWP increased > 7 mmHg or CVP increased > 4 mmHg.
- Repeat challenge if PAWP increased < 3 mmHg or CVP increased < 2 mmHg.
- Observe patient for 10 minutes and re-profile if PAWP increased > 3 mmHg but < 7 mmHg or CVP increased > 2 mmHg or <4 mmHg.
- Observe SVI and RVEDVI if RV volume values are available.
- Discontinue challenge if:
  SVI fails to increase by at least 10 % and RVEDVI increases by 25% or
  RVEDVI is > 140 ml/m2 and PAWP increases > 7 mmHg.

Optional Baseline RVEDVI Value Guidelines:

- If RVEDVI < 90 ml/m2 or mid range 90- 140 ml/m2, administer fluid challenge.

- If RVEDVI > 140 ml/m2, do not administer fluid.

Central Venous Catheter (CVC) Infusion Rates

7F Double Lumen and Triple Lumen Polyurethane Multi-Med Catheters

CATHETER	AVERAGE PERFORMANCE FLOW RATE		
	16 CM LONG (ML/HR)	20 CM LONG (ML/HR)	CROSS-SECTION GAUGE EQUIVALENCE
Triple Lumen			
Proximal	1670	1420	18
Medial	1500	1300	18
Distal	3510	3160	16
Double Lumen			
Proximal	3620	3200	16
Distal	3608	3292	16

*References differ on PAWP and CVP ranges.

Swan-Ganz Catheter Reference Charts

The chart below describes the wide breath of line of the Swan-Ganz catheters manufactured by Baxter Edwards Critical-Care Division.

CATHETER NAME	MODEL NUMBER	PAP/ PAWP	PROX./ RA	BCO	CCO
Base TD	131HF7	•	•	•	
VIP	831HF75	•	•	•	
VIP+	93A-834H-F7.5	•	•	•	
Paceport	93A-931H-F7.5	•	•	•	
AV Paceport	93A-991H-8F	•	•	•	
Pacing TD	93-200H-7F	•	•	•	
Bipolar Pacing	97-130-5F				
Bipolar Pacing	97-120-5F				
VIP Bipolar Pacing	97- K140H-5F				
CCO	139H-7.5F	•	•		•
CCOmbo	744H-7.5F	•	•		•
CCOmbo/VIP	746H-8F	•	•		•
CCOmbo/EDV	757HF8	•	•		•
SvO2	741HF75	•	•		
SvO2/Paceport	780HF75	•	•		
RVEDV/EF	431H-7.5F 434H-7.5F 435H-7.5F	•	•	•	
REF/Ox	750H-7.5F 754H-7.5F 759HF75	•	•	•	
REF/Ox/Paceport	791HF8	•	•	•	
Monitoring Catheters Double lumen	93-110-5F 93-123-6F	•			
Triple lumen Monitoring	93-114-7F 93-115-7F	•	•		
Pediatric Double Lumen Monitoring	93-116-4F 93-117-5F	•			
Pediatric Thermodilution	93-132-5F	•	•	•	
Adults with Small Vessels Thermodilution	93A-096-6F	•	•	•	
Base TD Hi-Shore	93A-141H-7F	•	•	•	
Base TD S-Tip	151-7F	•	•	•	
CardioCath	93A-143HT-7F	•	•	•	
ControlCath	C144-7F	•	•		
ControlCath S tip	S144H-7F	•	•		
Small French Oximetry	94-040-4F				
Pulmonary Angiography	93A-191H-7F				

This chart can be used as a quick ready reference guide to choose a catheter specific to the needs of the patient.

VIP PORTS	SVO2	RVEDV /EF	PACING	ADDITIONAL SPECIFICATIONS/COMMENTS
				With/Without Heparin, proximal injectate port 30 cm
•				With/Without Heparin proximal injectate port 30 cm, RA infusion port at 31 cm
•				RA infusion port 31 cm, injectate port 30 cm, RV infusion port 19 cm
•			•	Injectate port 30 cm, RV pacing or infusion port 19 cm
			•	Injectate port 30 cm, RA pacing or infusion port 27 cm, RV pacing or infusion port 19 cm
			•	Injectate port 30 cm; A, V, or A-V Pacing
			•	IVC/With or W/O insertion Kit, femoral approach
			•	SVC/With or W/O insertion kit
			•	Venous infusion port 12 cm
				Continuous cardiac output
	•			CCO/Sv02
•	•			CCO/Sv02/VIP Port
•	•	•		CCO/Sv02/EDV
	•			Continuous mixed venous oxygen saturation monitoring
	•		•	RV pacing or infusion port 19 cm
•	•		•	Infusion port 31 cm, injectate ports at 21 or 24 cm depending on model, with or without intracardiac electrodes
•	•	•		Infusion port 31 cm, injectate ports at 21 or 24 cm depending on model, with or without intracardiac electrodes
	•	•	•	Additional RV Pacing or infusion lumen at 19 cm
				Available in S-Tip or T-Tip configuration
				Proximal infusion port 30 or 20 cm
				60 cm in length
				75 cm in length, injectate port 15 cm
				110 cm in length, injectate port 30 cm
				Stiffer design for maneuverability
				Pre-molded "S" bend for facilitating femoral approaches
				Cath lab use, femoral approach
				Cath lab use, C shaped tip for femoral or SVC approach
				Cath lab use, S shaped tip for femoral approach
	•			Small french oximetry catheters for regional oxygen saturation monitoring.
				Available with or without heparin.

Standard Pulmonary Artery Catheter: General Indications

The pulmonary artery catheter is designed for measuring intra-cardiac and pulmonary artery pressures. Catheters with a thermistor near the distal tip can be used to measure cardiac output with the thermodilution method. Additionally, mixed venous saturation (SvO_2) values can be obtained from blood samples taken from the distal tip which lies in the pulmonary artery. The SvO_2 value then can be used in additional oxygenation utilization parameters.

General indications for use include obtaining information to make diagnosis, observing response to interventions and therapies and providing continuous monitoring of the patient's condition. Patients who are hemodynamically unstable may require closer monitoring of their cardiovascular status.

General indications for using the pulmonary artery catheter have been defined for patients in cardiac surgery. They include:

Patients undergoing coronary artery bypass grafts, who have:

• Poor left ventricular function; LVEDP > 18 mmHg; LVEF < 40 %

• LV wall motion abnormalities

• Recent MI (less than 6 months) or complications of MI

• Severe pre-operative angina

• Greater than 75% left main coronary artery disease

Patients with:

• Valvular disease

• Pulmonary hypertension

• Complex cardiac lesions

• Combined cardiac and valve procedures

• Over 65 years old

• Concomitant systemic diseases

Adapted from: Hensley FA, Martin DE (eds). *A Practical Approach to Cardiac Anesthesia* 2nd Ed. Boston: Little, Brown and Co. 1995.

Standard Pulmonary Artery Catheter: General Indications (continued)

Recent controversies regarding the use of the pulmonary artery catheter in the critical care arena prompted the organization of the Pulmonary Artery Catheter Consensus Conference. The participants of the conference examined important issues related to the indications and clinical use of the PAC by performing a review of the literature. Diseases or disorders investigated are listed below.

Cardiovascular Disease
• Myocardial infarction with; hypotension or cardiogenic shock, mechanical complications, or right ventricular infarction

• Congestive heart failure

• Pulmonary hypertension

• Shock or hemodynamic instability

Perioperative Period
• Cardiac surgery; high risk

• Peripheral vascular surgery; (reduced complications, reduced mortality)

• Aortic surgery; low or high risk

• Neurosurgery

• Trauma

Sepsis/Septic Shock

Supranormal Oxygen Delivery;
• SIRS, High - risk surgery

Respiratory Failure

Pediatric Patients (certain patients and conditions)

Adapted from: Controversies in Pulmonary Artery Catheterization. Pulmonary Artery Catheter Consensus Statement. New Horizons 1997.: 175-194.

General Indications:
Base Thermodilution Model 131

1. Assessment of a patient's hemodynamic condition through direct intracardiac and pulmonary artery pressure monitoring.

2. Assessment of oxygen delivery parameters through intermittent determination of cardiac output by bolus thermodilution.

3. Assessment of oxygen utilization parameters through sampling of mixed venous blood from distal lumen in the pulmonary artery.

Catheters may have AMC THROMBOSHIELD, an optional antimicrobial coating that decreases viable microbe counts on the surface of the catheter during handling and placement.

Note: Catheter markings occur every 10 cm. Identification of lumen exits are measured from the distal tip; i.e., proximal lumen is 30 cm form the distal tip.

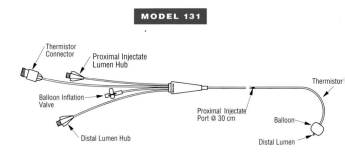

MODEL 131

Thermistor Connector

Proximal Injectate Lumen Hub

Balloon Inflation Valve

Distal Lumen Hub

Proximal Injectate Port @ 30 cm

Thermistor

Balloon

Distal Lumen

Venous Infusion Catheters:
Models 831 and 834

Venous Infusion Catheters provide additional lumens that exit either in the RA or both RA and RV, depending on the type of catheter. Clinical indications include those when central circulation access is needed for multiple volume and solution infusions at a high flow rate. Intra-atrial or intra-ventricular pressure monitoring can also be obtained with these additional lumens.

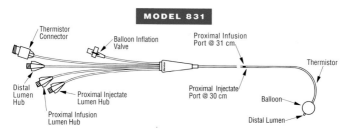

Additional right atrial lumen exists at 31 cm from the tip for fluid infusion or pressure monitoring.

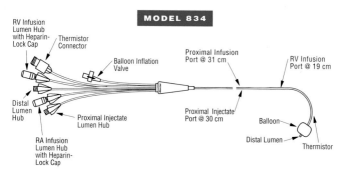

Additional RA lumen and RV lumen exits at 19 cm from tip to assure precise RV pressure monitoring.

Paceport Catheters:
Models 931 Paceport and 991 A-V Paceport

In addition to traditional hemodynamic monitoring, the Paceport catheters provide either ventricular pacing, atrial or atrio-ventricular pacing on demand. Clinical conditions include those in which managing the patient's ventricular heart rate is needed or optimizing cardiac output with synchronized AV pacing is required. Patients with known LBBB may be at risk for developing a complete heart block during PAC insertion. The Paceport catheter provides for rapid ventricular pacing if this occurs and the patient requires hemodynamic monitoring.

Temporary atrial, ventricular or atrioventricular pacing can be instituted with the use of the Chandler Transluminal V-Pacing Probe and atrial J pacing probe.

The additional lumens (RV lumen exits at 19 cm from the tip, RA exits at 27 cm) can also be used for pressure monitoring of their respective chambers or for additional fluid infusions.

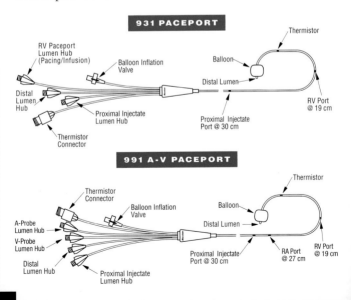

Pacing Probes 100 and 500

The 98-100H Chandler Transluminal V-Pacing Probe can be used for standby ventricular pacing when the patient's condition warrants. When the probe is not inserted, the lumen that exits at 19 cm from the distal tip may be used for RV pressure monitoring or infusion of fluids or solutions.

These probes can also be used for intra-atrial or ventricular ECG monitoring.

The Flex-Tip Transluminal A-Pacing probe (model 98-500H) can be inserted into the A-Probe lumen of the A-V Paceport catheter for atrial pacing. The lumen exits at 27 cm from the distal tip.

For atrio-ventricular pacing, the 991H is used with both the 98-100H Chandler V-Pacing probe and the 98-500H. Clinical indications include patients who would benefit from AV sequential pacing for optimization of cardiac output.

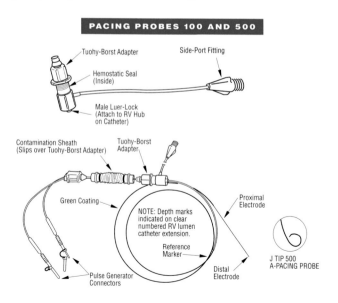

PACING PROBES 100 AND 500

Tuohy-Borst Adapter

Side-Port Fitting

Hemostatic Seal (Inside)

Male Luer-Lock (Attach to RV Hub on Catheter)

Contamination Sheath (Slips over Tuohy-Borst Adapter)

Tuohy-Borst Adapter

Green Coating

NOTE: Depth marks indicated on clear numbered RV lumen catheter extension.

Proximal Electrode

Reference Marker

Distal Electrode

Pulse Generator Connectors

J TIP 500 A-PACING PROBE

Pacing TD 200 and 205

Atrial and ventricular pacing electrodes are placed on the catheter to provide on-demand atrial, ventricular or AV sequential pacing. The 205 catheter is designed for patients with smaller anatomy to enhance capture for pacing. This catheter satisfies pacing indications previously stated with Paceport.

Temporary atrial, ventricular or atrioventricular pacing can be instituted rapidly. Intra-atrial and intra-ventricular ECG monitoring can be obtained without electro-cautery interference during surgery which is invaluable in triggering intra-aortic balloon pumps.

PACING TD 200

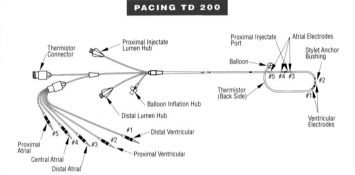

CCO 139

Continuous Cardiac Output Catheters

Catheters modified with a thermal filament and combined with the Vigilance Monitoring System can provide cardiac output measurements automatically on a continuous basis. Patients who would benefit from CCO monitoring include those requiring close monitoring of their cardiovascular status and their response to interventions and fluid. Additionally, since the cardiac output values are obtained without a manual injectate, both fluid restricted and immunocompromised patients may not be placed at risk of fluid overload or infection.

CCO 139

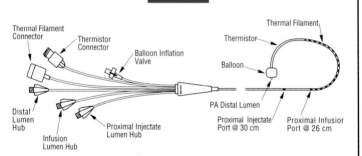

Thermal Filament Connector
Thermistor Connector
Balloon Inflation Valve
Distal Lumen Hub
Infusion Lumen Hub
Proximal Injectate Lumen Hub
Thermal Filament
Thermistor
Balloon
PA Distal Lumen
Proximal Injectate Port @ 30 cm
Proximal Infusion Port @ 26 cm

SvO₂ 741

Oximetry Catheters

The family of catheters that contain fiberoptics for mixed venous oxygen saturation monitoring provides continuous SvO₂ monitoring. Clinical indications include patient conditions where the balance between oxygen delivery and demand needs to be assessed. The SvO₂ value can be used to further assess the oxygen utilization indices for the critically ill patient. Additionally, the SvO₂ value has been used to diagnose the presence of intracardiac shunts. The Paceport Oximetry TD catheter is intended for use in patients who require hemodynamic monitoring when temporary transvenous pacing is anticipated.

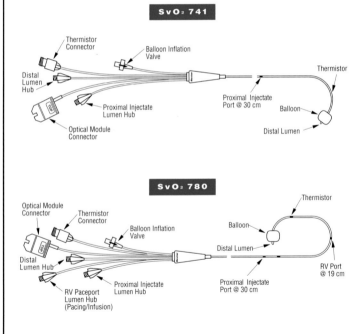

SvO₂ 741

Thermistor Connector

Balloon Inflation Valve

Thermistor

Distal Lumen Hub

Proximal Injectate Port @ 30 cm

Proximal Injectate Lumen Hub

Balloon

Optical Module Connector

Distal Lumen

SvO₂ 780

Optical Module Connector

Thermistor Connector

Balloon Inflation Valve

Thermistor

Balloon

Distal Lumen

Distal Lumen Hub

RV Port @ 19 cm

RV Paceport Lumen Hub (Pacing/Infusion)

Proximal Injectate Lumen Hub

Proximal Injectate Port @ 30 cm

CCOmbo/VIP: 744 and 746

By combining two continuous assessment technologies in one catheter, CCO and SvO₂ can be provided to the clinician on an automatic basis. Patients who require close observation of their cardiovascular status may benefit from these catheters.

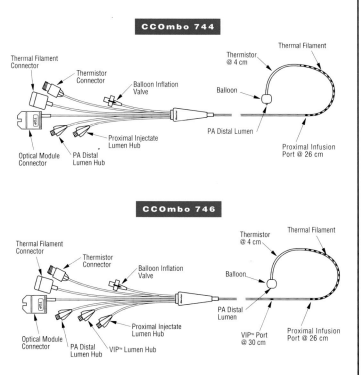

CCOmbo 744

Thermal Filament Connector
Thermistor Connector
Balloon Inflation Valve
Optical Module Connector
PA Distal Lumen Hub
Proximal Injectate Lumen Hub

Thermistor @ 4 cm
Thermal Filament
Balloon
PA Distal Lumen
Proximal Infusion Port @ 26 cm

CCOmbo 746

Thermal Filament Connector
Thermistor Connector
Balloon Inflation Valve
Optical Module Connector
PA Distal Lumen Hub
VIP™ Lumen Hub
Proximal Injectate Lumen Hub

Thermistor @ 4 cm
Thermal Filament
Balloon
PA Distal Lumen
VIP™ Port @ 30 cm
Proximal Infusion Port @ 26 cm

RV Volumetrics: 431

Volumetric Catheters

Catheters that have a fast response thermistor and are attached to a special computer can measure the right ventricular ejection fraction. Other parameters obtained include: right ventricular end-diastolic volume (RVEDV), right ventricular end-systolic volume (RVESV) and stroke volume (SV). Volumetric data have been shown to provide a more precise assessment of the volume status of the patient rather than the use of pressure based indices alone. Indications for use of the volumetric catheter include conditions in which volume resuscitation is required and fluid shifts occur. In addition, patients with the possibility of right ventricular failure may benefit from use of this catheter.

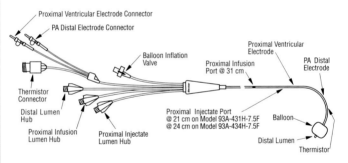

RV VOLUMETRICS 431

Proximal Ventricular Electrode Connector
PA Distal Electrode Connector
Balloon Inflation Valve
Proximal Ventricular Electrode
PA Distal Electrode
Proximal Infusion Port @ 31 cm
Thermistor Connector
Distal Lumen Hub
Proximal Infusion Lumen Hub
Proximal Injectate Lumen Hub
Proximal Injectate Port @ 21 cm on Model 93A-431H-7.5F @ 24 cm on Model 93A-434H-7.5F
Balloon
Distal Lumen
Thermistor

REF/Ox and REF/Ox Pacing: 758, 759, 791

These catheters provide right ventricular volumetric data as well as SvO₂ on a continuous basis. When used with the Explorer Computer system, dual oximetry assessment variables such as O2EI and VQI can be displayed. Right ventricular pacing can be obtained with use of the 791 or 794 catheter model.

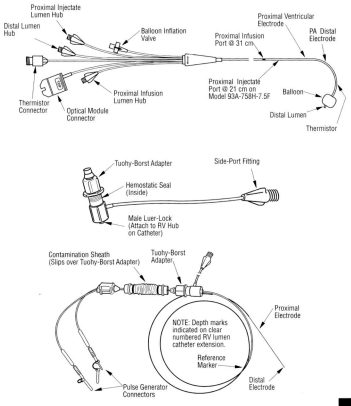

CCOmbo/EDV: 757

The CCOmbo/EDV catheter can be used for patients who require continuous assessment of their cardiac output and mixed venous oxygen saturation values, as well as more precise assessment of their preload status.

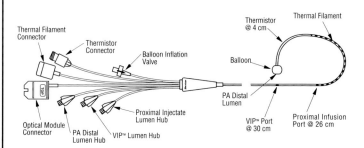

RV VOLUMETRICS CCOmbo 757

Thermal Filament Connector

Thermistor Connector

Balloon Inflation Valve

Optical Module Connector

PA Distal Lumen Hub

VIP™ Lumen Hub

Proximal Injectate Lumen Hub

Thermistor @ 4 cm

Thermal Filament

Balloon

PA Distal Lumen

VIP™ Port @ 30 cm

Proximal Infusion Port @ 26 cm

General Catheter Specifications

Most models of Swan-Ganz catheters have certain specifications that are common to all. Below is a listing of common catheter specifications. Specific specifications can be found on the product information sheet. Different manufacturers of thermodilution PA catheters may have different specifications and should be noted.

Color Body	Yellow
Usable Length (cm)	110
French Size	Varies with catheter model
Introducer Size Required	Varies with catheter model
Balloon Diameter	
Inflated (mm)	13
Deflated (F)	8
Balloon Inflation Syringe	3cc, limited to 1.5cc
Thermistor Nominal Resistance (+/- 15% @ 37°C ohms)	14,004
Resistance Rate Change (ohms/°C)	520
Thermistor Location	4 cm from tip
Nominal 63% Thermistor Response Time	95 milliseconds
Blood Temperature Measurement Accuracy	17°C-31°C+/-0.5°C 31°C-43°C+/-0.3°C

Selected Catheter Specifications

MODEL NUMBERS	131	831/834	931/991	139	741/780	744/746
DISTANCE FROM TIP PORT EXITS (CM)						
Proximal Injectate	30	30	30	26	30	26
Proximal Infusion		31	NA/27	30		NA/30
RV Infusion		NA/19	19		NA/19	
Thermal Filament				14 - 25		14 - 25
LUMEN VOLUME (ML)						
PA/Distal	1.02	0.91	0.87/0.93	0.9		0.96/0.90
Proximal Injectate	0.81	0.76/0.75	0.94/0.70	0.8		0.95/0.85
Proximal Infusion		0.95/0.97	NA/1.07	0.9		NA/1.10
RV Infusion/Pacing (without probe)	NA	NA/1.13				
INFUSION RATES (ML/HR)						
PA/Distal	425	280/324	291/324	250		320/325
Proximal Injectate	568	800/456	864/459	400		898/562
RA Infusion/Pacing		800/910	NA/66 with probe NA/811 without probe	800	NA	NA/988
RV Infusion/Pacing		NA/456	52/56 with probe 726/757 without probe		NA/53 with probe NA/759 without probe	
NATURAL FREQUENCY RESPONSE/ AMPLITUDE RATIO (HZ/AR)						
PA/Distal	37/3.0:1	34/2.4:1 33/2.6:1	32.2/2.5:1 31/2.4:1	25/ 2.0:1	32/2.5:1	25/2.1:1 26/2.1:1
Proximal Injectate	48 /3.3:1	48/2.9:1 37/2.4:1	46.6/2.8:1 44/2.7:1	33/ 2.5:1	41/2.8:1	45/2.7:1 40/2.6:1
Proximal Infusion		48/2.9:1 41/2.7:1	48/2.9:1 49/3.4:1	41/ 2.9:1		NA 40/2.5:1
RV Infusion/Pacing		NA 28/2.3:1	44.5/3.2:1 46/3.2:1		NA 44/3.2:1	

MODEL NUMBERS DISTANCE FROM TIP PORT EXITS (CM)	431/434 (435/439 ECG ELECTRODE FREE)	750/754 (758/759 ECG ELECTRODE FREE)	791/794	757
Proximal Injectate	21/24	21/24	21/24	26
Proximal Infusion	31	31	31	30
RV Infusion			19	
ECG Electrodes (cm)	6 and 16	6 and 16		Thermal Filament 14-25
LUMEN VOLUME (ML)				
PA/Distal	0.86/0.90	0.92	0.78	0.96
Proximal Injectate	0.93/0.91	0.98/0.96	0.87/0.86	0.85
Proximal Infusion	0.72/0.74	0.73	0.54	1.10
RV Infusion/Pacing			0.93 with probe 1.07 without probe	
INFUSION RATES (ML/HR)				
PA/Distal	294/321	320	238	325
Proximal Injectate	673/711	760/780	552/578	562
RA Infusion/ Pacing	431/462	440	145	988
RV Infusion/ Pacing			40 with probe 678 without probe	
NATURAL FREQUENCY RESPONSE/ AMPLITUDE RATIO (HZ/AR)				
PA/Distal	33/2.6:1 33/2.4:1	31/2.7:1	33.5/2.6:1	26/2.1:1
Proximal Injectate	44/3.1:1 43/3.0:1	41/3.1:1	35.2/2.7:1 36.6/2.6:1	40/2.6:1 40/2.5:1
Proximal Infusion	43/2.9:1 43/2.8:1		30.9/2.15:1	
RV Infusion/Pacing		43/3.0:1	47.1/3.8:1	

Adrenergic Receptors and Response to Activation

RECEPTOR	LOCATION	EFFECT
Alpha 1	Postsynaptic effector cells, primarily arterioles Coronary arterioles	Vasoconstriction
Alpha 2	Presynaptic membranes	Inhibition of norepinephrine release
Beta 1	Myocardial cells Sinoatrial node Atrioventricular junction	Increased contractility Increased automaticity Increased conductivity
Beta 2	Coronary arterioles Bronchioles	Vasodilation Bronchodilation
Dopamine 1	Renal and mesenteric arteries	Vasodilation Natriuresis
Dopamine 2	Presynaptic membrane	Inhibition of Norepinephrine release

TERMINOLOGY:

Automaticity: Impacts heart rate
Conductivity: Impacts conduction
Contractility: Impacts contraction
Chronotropy: Impacts heart rate
Inotropy: Impacts contractility
Dromotropy: Impacts conductivity

Notes:

Selected Cardiovascular Agents: Dosages and Responses

REFERENCE CHARTS

DRUG	ACTIONS:	DOSE RANGE
Amrinone (Inocor)	Phosphodiesterase inhibitor with strong vasodilation properties	IV loading dose: 0.75 mg/Kg over 3-5 min followed by a continuous infusion of 5-10 mcg/Kg/min. The bolus may be repeated in 30 minutes if required. The total daily dose should not exceed 10mcg/kg
Atropine Sulfate	Antiarrhythmic which directly blocks vagal effects on SA node	0.5 to 1 mg IV push. Repeat every 3 - 5 minutes. Maximum dose 0.03 to 0.04 mg/kg.
Digoxin	Cardiotonic glycoside. Increases inotrophism by promoting extracellular calcium to move to intercellular cytoplasm. Inhibits adenosine triphosphatase. Decreases conductivity through AV node.	Loading dose 0.5 to 1 mg IV or in divided doses P.O. over 24 hours. Maintenance dose 0.125 to 0.5 mg IV or PO daily 0.25 mg.
Dobutamine	Directly stimulates beta 1 receptors. Moderate stimulation of beta 2 receptors. Minimal stimulation of alpha receptors.	5- 15 mcg/Kg/min
Dopamine	Dopaminergic Effects: Renal, mesenteric vasodilatation. Beta Effects: Increased inotrophism Alpha Effects: Vasoconstriction	0.5 - 3mcg/Kg/min 5.0 - 10mcg/Kg/min > 10.0 mcg/Kg/min
Epinephrine	Low doses = Beta effect High doses = Alpha effect	0.005 - 0.02mcg/Kg/min 1mg or > IV push; 1 - 4 mcg/min infusion
Esmolol	Beta blocker	Loading dose 0.5 mg/Kg over 1 minute followed by infusion, titrate to desired effect: range 50 - 300 mcg/Kg/min
Phentolamine	Alpha blocker	IV bolus 5 - 15 mg. Infusion 0.2 - 1 mg/min
Propranolol	Beta blocker	IV bolus 1 - 3 mg in 50 ml NS or D5W slowly not to exceed 1 mg/min. Maintenance 10 - 80 mg PO t.i.d.or q.i.d.
Isoproterenol	Beta stimulator (B1 and B2)	2.0 - 20 mcg/min to achieve desired heart rate
Milrinone (Primacor)	Phophodiesterase inhibitor with less vasodilating properties than amrinone	Loading dose: 50 mcg/kg slowly over 10 minutes (undiluted) followed by continuous infusion 0.5mcg/Kg/min. Increase in increments of 0.375 mcg/Kg/min.
Neosynephrine	Alpha stimulator	0.10 - 0.18 mcg/min until BP stable, then 0.04 - 0.06 mg/min
Sodium Nitroprusside	Strong peripheral arterial vasodilator with lesser effects on the peripheral venous bed	0.25 - 10mcg/Kg/min
Nitroglycerin	Vasodilator with stronger effect on peripheral venous bed and coronary arteries than peripheral arterial bed	Start infusion @ 10mcg/min and increase in increments of 10mcg/min as needed to achieve desired effect
Norepinephrine	Low doses = Beta stimulation High doses = Alpha stimulation	Start at 0.05 - 0.1mcg/Kg/min and titrate up to 2.0 - 4.0 mcg/Kg/min
Verapamil	Calcium antagonist, combines arteriolar dilation and direct negative inotropic effect.	2.5 to 5.0 mg IV bolus over 1-2 minutes. Repeat 5-10 mg in 15 to 30 minutes. Maximum dose: 30 mg.

Chart compiled from references: 7,8,18,23. Effects noted may vary according to reference.
Caution: Please refer to current product package inserts for indications, contraindications, precautions and instructions for use.

HR	MAP	CO	PAWP	SVR	PVR	NOTES
O/↑	O/↑	↑	↓	↓	↓	ACLS Guidelines state optimal use requires hemodynamic monitoring.
↑	↑	↑	O	O	O	
O/↓	O/↑	↑	O/↓	O	O	Hemodynamic response depends on patient condition.
O/↑	↑	↑	↓	↓	↓	ACLS Guidelines states hemodynamic monitoring is recommended for optimal use.
↑	↑	↑	↓	↑	O	Use in hypovolemic patient only after fluid resuscitation.
↑	↑	↑	↑	↑	↑	
↓	↓	O/↓	O/↑	↓	↓	
↑	↑	↑	↓	↑	O/↑	In low output LV failure, large doses are required. Also used in hypertensive crisis.
↓	↓	↓	↓	O	↑	
↑	↑	↑	↓	↓	↓	
↓	↓	↑	↓	↓	↓	
O	↓	↑	↓	↓	↓	
O	↓	O/↑	↓	↓	↓	
↓	↓	O	↓	↓	↓	Second drug of choice for PSVT. Peripheral vasodilation produces BP drop.

Typical Hemodynamic Profiles in Various Acute Conditions

CONDITION	HR	MAP	CO/CI	CVP/RAP	PAP/PAWP	NOTES
Left Ventricular Failure	↑	↓	↓	↑	↑	
Pulmonary Edema (Cardiogenic)	↑	N, ↓	↓	↑	↑PAWP > 25 mmHg	
Massive Pulmonary Embolism	↑	↓V	↓	↑	↑PAD > PAWP by >5 mmHg	↑PVR
Acute Ventricular Septal Defect	↑	↓	↓	↑	↑giant "v" wave on PAWP tracing	O_2 step up noted in SvO_2
Acute Mitral Valve Regurgitation	↑	↓	↓	↑	↑giant "v" waves on PAWP tracing	No O_2 step up noted in SvO_2
Cardiac Tamponade	↑	↓	↓	↑	↑CVP, PAD and PAW equalized	↓RVEDVI
Right Ventricular Failure	↑,V	↓,V	↓	↑	PAP ↑, PAWP N/↓/↓	↑RVEDVI
Hypovolemic Shock	↑	↓	↓	↓	↓	↑Oxygen extraction ↑SVR
Cardiogenic Shock	↑	↓	↓	↑	↑	↑Oxygen extraction ↑SVR
Septic Shock	↑	↓	↑,↓	↓,↑	↓,↑	SVR changes, ↓Oxygen extraction ↓SVR

↑ = Increased, ↓ = Decreased, N= Normal, V=Varies

Chart compiled from references: 8,18,23, 30.

Indications For Hemodynamic Monitoring
Pulmonary Artery Catheterization

ACC/AHA American College of Cardiology and American Heart Association, ACP American College of Physicians, ASA American Society of Anesthesiologists, ESICM European Society of Intensive Care Medicine   *Modified listing

CLINICAL INDICATIONS	ACC/AHA	ACP	ASA	ESICM
Establish or assist in establishing a "specific" diagnosis	*	*		*
VSD vs AMR in AMI	*	*		*
RVI in selected patients with IWMI	*	*		*
Evaluate severity of pulmonary embolism	*	*		*
Differentiate between types of shock states	*	*		*
Differentiate between causes of pulmonary edema (cardiogenic vs non-cardiogenic)	*	*		*
Help direct management of medical patients in whom knowledge of intravascular pressures and flow will alter treatment when clinical estimates (e.g. bedside examination, chest x-ray, or fluid challenge) are not reliable.	*	*		*
Complex cardiac conditions; hypotension unresponsive to fluid challenge, marked hemodynamic instability requiring vasoactive drugs	*	*		*
Monitor response and guide therapy with fluids, diuretics, inotropes, or positive pressure ventilation	*	*	*	*
Perioperative monitoring in high risk patients	*	*	*	*
Clinical Investigation Tool: Developing new concepts Assessing prognostic subsets Assessing hemodynamic responses to new therapies	* * * *	* * * *		* * * *

Recommendations for Balloon Flotation Right-Heart Catheter Monitoring (AHA/ACC)

Class I
1. Severe or progressive CHF or pulmonary edema.
2. Cardiogenic shock or progressive hypotension.
3. Suspected mechanical complications of acute infarction; i.e., VSD, papillary muscle rupture or pericardial tamponade.

Class IIa
1. Hypotension that does not respond promptly to fluid administration in a patient without pulmonary congestion.

Class III
1. Patients with acute infarction without evidence of cardiac or pulmonary complications.

Recommendations for Intra-arterial Pressure Monitoring

Class I
1. Patients with severe hypotension (systolic arterial pressure less than 80 mm Hg) and/or cardiogenic shock.
2. Patients receiving vasopressor agents.

Class IIa
1. Patients receiving intravenous sodium nitroprusside or other potent vasodilators.

Class IIb
1. Hemodynamically stable patients receiving intravenous nitroglycerin for myocardial ischemia.
2. Patients receiving intravenous inotropic agents.

Class III
1. Patients with acute infarction who are hemodynamically stable.

Killip Classification of Heart Failure in Acute Myocardial Infarction

CLASS	CLINICAL SIGNS	MORTALITY
I	No signs of congestive heart failure	6 %
II	Mild or moderate heart failure: rales heard over as much as 50% of bilateral lung fields	17 %
III	Pulmonary edema: rales heard > 50% bilateral lung fields	38 %
IV	Cardiogenic shock: BP< 90 mmHg; signs of inadequate peripheral perfusion including reduced UO, cold & clammy skin, cyanosis, mental obtundation	81 %

Source: Killip T and Kimball JT. Am J Cardiol 20:457, 1967.

New York Heart Classification of Cardiovascular Disease

CLASS	SUBJECTIVE ASSESSMENT	PROGNOSIS
I	Normal cardiac output without systemic or pulmonary congestion; asymptomatic at rest and on heavy exertion	Good
II	Normal cardiac output maintained with a moderate increase in pulmonary-systemic congestion; symptomatic on exertion	Good with therapy
III	Normal cardiac output maintained with a marked increase in pulmonary-systemic congestion; symptomatic on mild exercise	Fair with therapy
IV	Cardiac output reduced at rest with a marked increase in pulmonary - systemic congestion; symptomatic at rest	Guarded despite therapy

Source: Killip T and Kimball JT. Am J Cardiol 20:457, 1967.

American College of Cardiology Clinical & Hemodynamic Classes of AMI

LEVEL	CLASSIFICATION	CARDIAC INDEX L/M/M²	PAWP mmHg	BP mmHg
I Rx	No pulmonary congestion IV NTG to modify mortality, infarct size and pain	2.7 +/- 0.5	</= 12	NL
II Rx	Isolated pulmonary congestion IV NTG, diuretics (↓ preload), morphine	>3.0	>12	↑
III Rx	Isolated peripheral hypotension Careful hydration (↑ PAWP to 18)	<2.7	<9	↓
IV Rx	Both pulmonary congestion and peripheral hypotension Mild LV failure Severe LV failure Combined use Dopamine & dobutamine (or Amrinone) consider IABP	 <2.5 <1.8	 >18< 22 >22	 NL ↑,↓
V Rx	Cardiogenic shock PTCA or CABG and circulatory support	<1.8	>18	↓
VI Rx	Shock secondary to RV infarction Volume and inotropes to support circulation	<1.8	<18	↓

Source: J Am Coll Cardiol 16:249 1990.

Forrester Classification Hemodynamic Subsets of Acute Myocardial Infarction

SUBSET CLINICAL DESCRIPTION	CARDIAC INDEX L/MIN/M2	PAWP mmHg	THERAPY	MORTALITY %
I No Failure	> 2.2	< 18	Sedate	3
II Pulmonary Congestion	> 2.2	>18	Normal BP: Diuretics ↑BP: Vasodilators	9
III Peripheral Hypotension	< 2.2	<18	↑HR: Add volume ↓HR: Pacing	23
IV Congestion & Hypoperfusion	< 2.2	> 18	↓BP: Inotropes Normal BP: Vasodilators	51

Compiled from references: 13, 17, 29.

Glasgow Coma Scale

NEUROLOGICAL FUNCTION:		POINTS
Eye Opening	Spontaneous	4
	To sound	3
	To pain	2
	Never	1
Best Motor Response	Obeys commands	6
	Localizes pain	5
	Flexion (withdraws)	4
	Flexion (abnormal)	3
	Extension	2
Best Verbal Response	Oriented	5
	Confused conversation	4
	Inappropriate words	3
	Incomprehensible sounds	2
	None	1

Source: Wilkinson HA: Neurologic monitoring in the intensive care unit in *Intensive Care Medicine*, ed. J.M Rippe et al., Boston, Little, Brown and Company, 1985, p. 1032.

The APACHE II Severity of Disease Classification System

	HIGH ABNORMAL RANGE				0	LOW ABNORMAL RANGE			
	+4	+3	+2	+1	0	+1	+2	+3	+4
TEMPERATURE – rectal (°C)	≥41°	39	-40.9°	38.5°-38.9°	36°-38.4°	34°-35.9°	32°-33.9°	30°-31.9°	≤29.9°
MEAN ARTERIAL PRESSURE – mm Hg	≥160	130-159	110-129		70-109		50-69		≤49
HEART RATE (ventricular response)	≥180	140-179	110-139		70-109		55-69	40-54	≤39
RESPIRATORY RATE (non-ventilated or ventilated)	≥50	35-49		25-34	12-24	10-11	6-9		≤5
OXYGENATION A-aDO2 or PaO2 (mm Hg) a. FIO2 ≥ 0.5 record A-aDO2	≥500	350-499	200-349		<200				
b. FIO2 ≤ 0.5 record only PaO2					PO2≥7	PO2 61-70		PO2 55-60	PO2≤55
ARTERIAL pH	≥7.7	7.6-7.69		7.5-7.59	7.33-7.49		7.25-7.32	7.15-7.24	<7.15
SERUM SODIUM (mmol/L)	≥180	160-179	155-159	150-154	130-149		120-129	111-119	≤110
SERUM POTASSIUM (mmol/L)	≥7	6-6.9		5.5-5.9	3.5-5.4	3-3.4	2.5-2.9		<2.5
SERUM CREATININE (mg/100 ml) (Double point score for acute renal failure)	≥3.5	2-3.4	1.5-1.9		0.6-1.4		<0.6		
HEMATOCRIT (%)	≥60		50-59.9	46-49.9	30-45.9		20-29.9		<20
WHITE BLOOD COUNT (total/mm3) (in 1,000s)	≥40		20-39.9	15-19.9	3-14.9		1-2.9		<1
GLASGOW COMA SCALE (GCS) Score = 15 minus actual GCS									
A Total ACUTE PHYSIOLOGY SCORE (APS): Sum of the 12 individual variable points									
Serum HCO₃ (venous-mmol/L) [Not preferred, use if no ABGs]	≥52	41-51.9		32-40.9	22-31.9		18-21.9	15-17.9	<15

B **Age Points:** Assign points to age as follows: Age(yrs)Points

<44	0
45-54	2
55-64	3
65-74	5
>75	6

C **Chronic Health Points**

If the patient has a history of severe organ system insufficiency or is immunocompromised, assign points as follow:
a. for nonoperative or emergency postoperative patients – 5 points or
b. for elective postoperative patient – 2 points

Definitions

Organ insufficiency or immunocompromised state must have been evident prior to this hospital admission and conform to the following criteria:

Liver:

Biopsy-proven cirrhosis and documented portal hypertension; episodes of past upper GI bleeding attributed to portal hypertension; or prior episodes of hepatic failure/encephalopathy/coma.

Cardiovascular: New York Heart Association Class IV.

Respiratory:

Chronic restrictive, obstructive, or vascular disease resulting in severe exercise restriction, i.e., unable to climb stairs or perform household duties; or documented chronic hypoxia, hypercapnia, secondary polycythemia, severe pulmonary hypertension (>40 mm Hg), or respiratory dependency.

Renal: Receiving chronic dialysis.

Immunocompromised: Immunosuppression, chemotherapy, radiation, long-term or recent high-dose steroids, or has a disease that is sufficiently advanced to suppress resistance to infection, e.g., leukemia, lymphoma, AIDS.

APACHE II Score

Sum of A + B + C

A APS points
B Age points
C Chronic Health points
Total **Apache II**

Source: Knaus, W.A. et al: APACHE II: A severity of disease classification system, *Crit. Care Med.* 13(10):818-829, 1985.

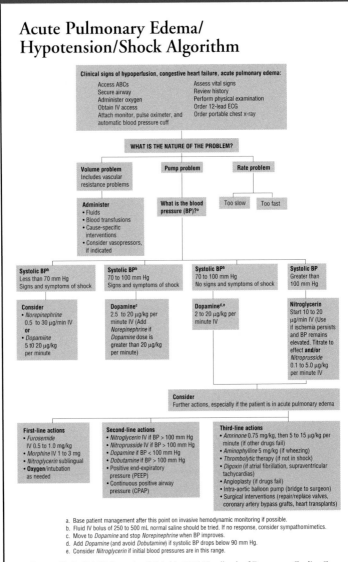

Acute Pulmonary Edema/ Hypotension/Shock Algorithm

Clinical signs of hypoperfusion, congestive heart failure, acute pulmonary edema:

Access ABCs
Secure airway
Administer oxygen
Obtain IV access
Attach monitor, pulse oximeter, and automatic blood pressure cuff

Assess vital signs
Review history
Perform physical examination
Order 12-lead ECG
Order portable chest x-ray

WHAT IS THE NATURE OF THE PROBLEM?

Volume problem
Includes vascular resistance problems

Pump problem

Rate problem

Administer
• Fluids
• Blood transfusions
• Cause-specific interventions
• Consider vasopressors, if indicated

What is the blood pressure (BP)?[a]

Too slow   Too fast

Systolic BP[b]
Less than 70 mm Hg
Signs and symptoms of shock

Systolic BP[b]
70 to 100 mm Hg
Signs and symptoms of shock

Systolic BP[b]
70 to 100 mm Hg
No signs and symptoms of shock

Systolic BP
Greater than 100 mm Hg

Consider
• *Norepinephrine* 0.5 to 30 µg/min IV
or
• *Dopamine* 5 to 20 µg/kg per minute

Dopamine[c]
2.5 to 20 µg/kg per minute IV (Add *Norepinephrine* if *Dopamine* dose is greater than 20 µg/kg per minute)

Dopamine[d,e]
2 to 20 µg/kg per minute IV

Nitroglycerin
Start 10 to 20 µg/min IV (Use if ischemia persists and BP remains elevated. Titrate to effect **and/or** *Nitroprusside* 0.1 to 5.0 µg/kg per minute IV

Consider
Further actions, especially if the patient is in acute pulmonary edema

First-line actions
• *Furosemide* IV 0.5 to 1.0 mg/kg
• *Morphine* IV 1 to 3 mg
• *Nitroglycerin* sublingual
• **Oxygen**/intubation as needed

Second-line actions
• *Nitroglycerin* IV if BP > 100 mm Hg
• *Nitroprusside* IV if BP > 100 mm Hg
• *Dopamine* if BP < 100 mm Hg
• *Dobutamine* if BP > 100 mm Hg
• Positive end-expiratory pressure (PEEP)
• Continuous positive airway pressure (CPAP)

Third-line actions
• *Amrinone* 0.75 mg/kg, then 5 to 15 µg/kg per minute (if other drugs fail)
• *Aminophylline* 5 mg/kg (if wheezing)
• *Thrombolytic* therapy (if not in shock)
• *Digoxin* (if atrial fibrillation, supraventricular tachycardias)
• Angioplasty (if drugs fail)
• Intra-aortic balloon pump (bridge to surgeon)
• Surgical interventions (repair/replace valves, coronary artery bypass grafts, heart transplants)

a. Base patient management after this point on invasive hemodynamic monitoring if possible.
b. Fluid IV bolus of 250 to 500 mL normal saline should be tried. If no response, consider sympathomimetics.
c. Move to *Dopamine* and stop *Norepinephrine* when BP improves.
d. Add *Dopamine* (and avoid *Dobutamine*) if BP drops below 90 mm Hg.
e. Consider *Nitroglycerin* if initial blood pressures are in this range.

Source: Hazinski MF, Cummins RO (eds). 1996 Handbook of Emergency Cardiac Care for Healthcare Providers. American Heart Association 1996.

Idealized Ventricular Function Curves

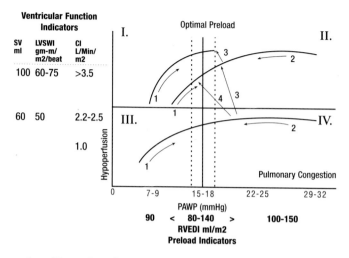

SV ml	LVSWI gm-m/ m2/beat	CI L/Min/ m2
100	60-75	>3.5
60	50	2.2-2.5
		1.0

I. **Normal Perfusion**
   No Pulmonary Congestion
II. **Normal Perfusion**
   Pulmonary Congestion
III. **Hypoperfusion**
   No Pulmonary Congestion
IV . **Hypoperfusion**
   Pulmonary Congestion

Possible Interventions

   1 = ↑ Preload; moves along same curve, volume

   2 = ↓ Preload; moves along same curve, diuretic/venodilator

   3 = ↑ Contractility; shifts to higher curve, minimal change in preload, positive inotrope

   4 = ↓ Afterload; shifts to a higher curve at a lower preload, afterload reducers, vasodilators

Chart compiled from references: 8,12,24,30.

Vigilance Monitor

Continuous Cardiac Output (CCO) and Mixed Venous Oxygen
Saturation (SvO₂)

To Begin SvO₂:

1. Connect catheter to optics module.
2. Press **SvO₂** on blue touch bar.
3. Select **IN VITRO CALIBRATION** on the touch bar.
4. Use the **CURSOR** key to select HGB (hemoglobin) **OR** Hct (hematocrit). Use default value or enter lab value using touch bar.
5. Press the **CAL** key.
6. Flush catheter; check balloon. Insert catheter in PA. **Press START SvO₂.**

To Invivo Calibrate SvO₂:

1. Press **SvO₂** on blue touch bar.
2. Press **INVIVO CALIBRATION**.
3. Press **DRAW**, after checking for SQI of 1 or 2.
4. Slowly waste discard, draw sample and send for analysis by co-oximeter.
5. Use the **CURSOR** to select value, enter lab results using touch bar.
6. Press **CAL**.

To Transport SvO₂:

1. After reconnecting patient cable and optics module, press **SvO₂** on touch bar.
2. Press **TRANSPORT**.
3. Press **RECALL**. *(Note: Calibration data must be less than 24 hours old.)*

To Begin CCO:

1. Connect thermal filament and thermistor connections on catheter to patient cable.

Vigilance Monitor (continued)

2. Press **START CCO** to begin Continuous Cardiac Output (CCO) monitoring.

To Configure Computer Screen (from Home Screen):

1. Press **SET UP** to change display format (temperature units, international units, time format, alarm volume, indexed/non-indexed values).
   - Press **CURSOR** to highlight format selection.
   - Once highlighted, press **CHANGE** to select desired parameters.
   - Press **HOME** to enter and return to home screen.

2. Press **ALARMS** to set alarms.
   - Press **ALARMS ON/OFF** to toggle the alarms suspended function.
   - Press **CCO** or **SvO₂** on the touch bar.
   - Press **HI/LOW** to set desired limit, and use touch bar to select value.
   - Press **HOME** to enter and return to home screen.

3. Press **TREND** to set trend time scale or to change graphic displays.
   - Use touch bar to select desired time interval from 30 minutes to 24 hours.
   - Press **EVENTS** to mark interventions. Use touch bar to select desired event.
   - Press **SELECT GRAPH** to set parameter and scale for Graph 1 or Graph 2.

(Note: CCO/CCI will be predetermined by selection in SET-UP.)

To Use Cardiac/Oxygen Profile:

1. Press **PATIENT DATA** to enter cardiac profile, which includes height/weight for BSA calculation (height and weight may be entered pre-insertion).
   - Press **EDIT** to input new values.
   - Press **CURSOR** to highlight desired parameter.
   - Use touch bar to enter new value.

Vigilance Monitor (continued)

- Press **CHANGE UNITS** while Height/Weight is highlighted to toggle between Metric/English units.
- Press **CALC** or **HOME** to calculate derived cardiac parameters.
- Press **OXYGEN PROFILE** to enter oxygen profile.
- Use **EDIT** and **CURSOR** keys to enter data.
- Press **CALC** to calculate derived oxygen parameters.
- Press **HOME** to return to home screen.

To Perform Bolus Cardiac Output:

1. Press **BOLUS CO** on touch bar.
2. Check **INJ VOL** (Injectate Volume) and **CATHETER** (Catheter Size) and **MODE** (automatic or manual). Use touch bar to change values.
3. Auto Mode: Begin injecting bolus within four (4) minutes after **INJECT** message.
   - Wait for CO to be displayed.
   - Inject subsequent boluses after **INJECT** message reappears.
   Manual Mode: Press **START** and inject bolus within 30 seconds
   - Wait for CO to be displayed.
   - Press start and inject subsequent boluses after **READY** message reappears.
4. Press **EDIT BOLUS** after desired number of boluses.
   - Use the touch bar to delete values from CO average. (Selecting twice will re-select value.)
   - Press **RETURN** after editing is completed.
   - Press **HOME** to return to home screen.
   - Press **START** to resume CCO.

To View Stat Mode (Fast Trend Estimates of CCO/CCI):

1. Press STAT on touch bar.
2. Ten boxes for CCO/CCI run data will appear. Most recent fast trend data will appear in top left box.

Vigilance Monitor (continued)

To Use Drug Calculation Mode:

1. Press **DRUG CALC** on touch bar when in the home screen.

2. If weight in data base it will be displayed on **Drug Calculation Screen.**

3. Enter data of highlighted parameter by using the numeric touchbar keys. Then Press **CURSOR**. Enter **Weight, Drug Quantity** and **Solution Volume**.

4. Entering **Drug Administration Rate** will automatically calculate **Infusion Rate**.

Note: Because of hard decimal point, at least a two digit entry is required. Examples: 5 mcg/kg/min=5.00 (3 digit entry); 1/2 mcg/kg/min=.50 (2 digit entry).

5. Entering **Infusion Rate** will automatically calculate **Drug Administration Rate**.

Refer to Vigilance Monitor Operator's Manual for detailed warnings, precautions and instructions for use.

Troubleshooting the CCOmbo Catheter

PROBLEM OR DISPLAYED MESSAGE	POSSIBLE CAUSE	SUGGESTED ACTION
CCO measurements do not agree with Bolus CO measurements	Catheter Position	Verify proper catheter position: Balloon inflation 1.25-1.5cc. Check for PAWP tracing. Transduce Injectate (RA/Blue) Lumen.
	Instrument Configuration	Verify that injectate volume and catheter size **OR** computation constant have been correctly selected.
	Faulty thermistor or injectate probe connection	Check injectate probe and catheter connection.
	Unstable baseline temperature affecting bolus CO measurements	Assess factors affecting PA temperature stability: rapid bolus infusions, shivering, patient movement, fighting ventilator. Wait 60 seconds between injections.
"Check Thermal Filament Position"	Flow around thermal filament may be reduced.	Verify proper catheter position. Verify free floating state of catheter.
"Warm Injectate" or "Injectate too Warm. Check Probe."	Injectate temperature within 8°C of blood temperature. Injectate temperature >30°C.	Use cooler injectate fluid: Maintain ice slush solution. If prefilled syringes, remove from cold source and use within 15 seconds. Check injectate probe connection. Replace injectate temperature probe.
"SQI = 4"	Catheter too distal. Low blood flow at catheter tip or catheter tip against vessel wall. Change in Hgb/Hct values. Catheter kinked or damaged.	Verify proper catheter position. Verify patency of catheter. Update Hgb/Hct values using **UPDATE** function. Check catheter for kinking and recalibrate. Replace catheter if required and recalibrate. After all above troubleshooting measures are utilized, press **OPTICAL RESET**
"Red/IR Transmit"	Optical Module contamination/Optical Module damage	Disconnect catheter from OM. Clean Optical connector on catheter and OM. Reconnect. If Error message disappears, do **INVIVO** call. If Error message remains, try different Optical Module. If Error message remains, change catheter.

Explorer Quick Reference Guide
6.37 Software

Initial Set-Up/In Vitro Calibration

1. Connect Optical module to machine, turn on Power
2. If "NEW PATIENT" option appears, Press
   "NEW PATIENT" Twice
3. Allow 20 minutes for optical module warm-up (5 minutes minum.)
4. Open 1st stage catheter packaging and connect catheter to
   optical module
5. Press "SvO$_2$"
6. Press "VITRO"
7. Input current "HGB" or "Hct" or use the displayed values
8. Press "CAL"
9. After "CAL OK" displayed, prepare catheter and insert
10. Press "OPERATE" after catheter is inserted.

In Vivo Calibration (Assess that "SQI" is under 4)

1. Press "SvO$_2$"
2. Press "VIVO"
3. Press "DRAW"
4. Draw discard slowly followed by lab samples (2cc/30 seconds)
5. After receiving lab values:
   Enter new "HGB" or "Hct", Press "ENTER"
   Enter new "SvO$_2$", Press "ENTER"
6. Press "CAL"

Update

1. Press "SvO$_2$"
2. Press "UPDATE"
3. Enter new "HGB" or "Hct", Press "ENTER"
4. Press "CAL"

Explorer Quick Reference Guide
6.37 Software (continued)

Cardiac Output/REF
1. Press "CO/REF"
2. Press "CC" (Check Computation Constant)
   Assess appropriate catheter model number
   Assess appropriate volume
   Connect appropriate temperature probe
3. Press "RETURN"
4. Press "START", Shoot output (REPEAT)
5. To average, Press "AVG"
   To delete any outputs, press "DELETE"
6. Enter the number(s) that corresponds to the cardiac output(s)
   to be deleted
7. Press "CALC"
8. Record Average Outputs
9. Press "MAIN" to return to Main Menu

BSA Entry
1. Press "SETUP" (Located above numeric key pad)
2. Press "DATA"
3. Enter Patient's "HEIGHT", Press "ENTER"
4. Enter Patient's "WEIGHT", Press "ENTER"
5. BSA will be calculated
6. Press "MAIN" to return to main menu

Patient Transport
Disconnect optical module connecting cable from Explorer Computer
(Do not disconnect catheter from optical module)

Refer to Explorer monitor operation manual for detailed warnings, precautions and
instructions for use.

Notes:

REF-1 Quick Reference Guide

1. Parameters Attained with REF-1

- CARDIAC OUTPUT (CO)=4 - 8.0 1/min
- CARDIAC INDEX (CI)=2.5 - 5.0 l/min/m2
- STROKE VOLUME(SV): The volume of blood ejected from the
  ventricle in each beat. SV=CO/HR x 1000
  Normal SV: 60 - 100 ml
  Normal SVI: 35 - 60 ml/m2
- END-DIASTOLIC VOLUME (EDV): The volume of blood in the
  ventricle at the end of the diastole. EDV = SV/EF
  Normal RV EDV: 100 - 160 ml
  Normal RV EDVI: 60 - 100 ml/m2
- END-SYSTOLIC VOLUME (ESV): The volume of blood in the
  ventricle at the end of systole. ESV = EDV - SV
  Normal RV ESV: 50 - 100 ml
  Normal RV ESVI: 30 - 60 ml/m2
- EJECTION FRACTION (EF): The percentage of blood ejected
  from the ventricle each beat.

$$EF = \frac{EDV\text{-}ESV}{EDV} \quad \text{or} \quad \frac{SV}{EDV}$$

Normal RVEF: 40 - 60%
*(NOTE: As with all measurements in hemodynamic monitoring, the
absolute number is not as important as trends and changes in response to
therapy.)*

2. Goal of RV Volumetric Measurements:

- Optimize RV Efficiency
- Optimize the Relationship Between EDV and SV
- **a.** In an efficient state, an increase in
  PRELOAD (EDV) will result
  in an INCREASE in STROKE
  VOLUME (SV).

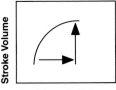

Stroke Volume

End-Diastolic Volume

REF-1 Quick Reference Guide (continued)

b. Prior to reaching the FLAT PART of the curve, an increase in PRELOAD (EDV) will increase SV while causing a decrease in Ejection Fraction.

c. On the FLAT PART of the curve, a further increase in PRELOAD (EDV) will not result in an increase in SV.

At this point, a further increase in volume may:

- Decrease oxygen supply
- Increase oxygen demand
- Decrease left ventricular compliance

Therapy should be directed at increasing contractility or reducing afterload.

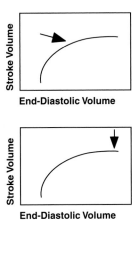

3. For the Hypotensive Patient:

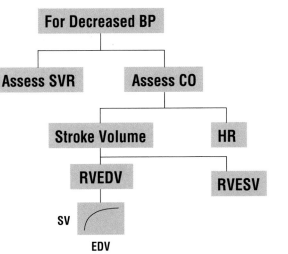

REF-1 Troubleshooting: Maximizing Accuracy and Reproducibility

1. Assess Catheter Location
• PROXIMAL INJECTATE PORT LOCATION:
  1 - 5 cm proximal to tricuspid valve.
  Before EF/CO determination, assess for appropriate
  PAWP waveform.
• THERMISTOR LOCATION:
  Before EF/CO determination, assess for appropriate
  PAWP waveform;
  Damped waveform should not be present.
  Balloon should require >1cc for inflation.
(If the PAWP is damped or if <1cc is required to inflate the balloon,
distal migration of the catheter may have occurred.)

2. Evaluate Technique
• Use of 5 or 10 cc iced injectate.
• Inject into blue Proximal Injectate lumen.
  NOTE: 10cc iced injectate is recommended for increased reproducibility.
• Check for appropriate computation constant.

COMPUTATION CONSTANTS (FOR 21 & 24 CM PORTS)

Volume	Injectate Temp (Iced Syringes) 0 -5(C	Co-Set 10 cc- 6 - 12(C 5 cc - 8 - 16(C
10cc	0.542	0.561
5 cc	0.247	0.259

• Smooth, rapid (10cc<4 sec) injection.
• Injection synchronized with end-expiration.
• For indexed values, verify that appropriate patient height
  and weight is entered.

3. Assess EF/CO Curve
• Check for rapid upstroke.
("Plateaus" on the curve may be seen
as the rapid response thermistor is
sensing the change in temperature
on a beat-to-beat basis.)
• Check for gradual return to baseline.

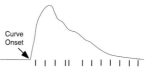
Curve Onset

QUICK REFERENCE GUIDES

REF-1 Troubleshooting: Maximizing Accuracy and Reproducibility (continued)

4. Observe Accuracy of the EKG Signal
• Observe the flashing green R-wave trigger light on the front of the REF-1.
• Compare the heart rate displayed on the prompt/trend display to the bedside monitor.

NOTE: For optimal EF values, the sensed HR from the REF-1 and the HR from the bedside monitor should be within two beats per minute.

• Observe the "tick" marks under the EF/CO curve.

(Tick marks under the curve should be regular and reflect the patient's heart rhythm.)

TO MAXIMIZE ACCURACY:
• Assess that all leads/connections are secure.
• Reposition reference lead.
• OPTION: Utilize SLAVE function: Disconnect intracardiac leads (cover with red caps) and reference lead and connect the EKG monitor signal (in lead II) to the EKG input on the rear of the REF-1™ using a $1/4$" stereo phone plug.

5. Assess Regularity of the EKG Signal
• Assess regularity of tick marks under the EF/CO curve.
• Assess that rhythm reflects patient's baseline.
• If irregular, repeat EF/CO determination when heart rate is stable/regular.
• If irregular, consider degree of irregularity and impact of irregularity on EF/CO determination.

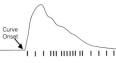
Curve Onset

6. Observe Accuracy of Paced Rhythm
• Evaluate EKG signal; assess for the presence of double sensing.

IN THE EVENT OF DOUBLE SENSING:
• Reposition leads to maximize either the atrial or ventricular spikes.
• Assess for appropriateness of mA levels.
• OPTION: Consider slaving from bedside monitor.

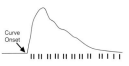
Curve Onset

Normal Hemodynamic Parameters – Adult

PARAMETER	EQUATION	NORMAL RANGE
Arterial Blood Pressure (BP)	Systolic (SBP) Diastolic (DBP)	90 - 140 mm Hg 60 - 90 mm Hg
Mean Arterial Pressure (MAP)	SBP+2DBP/3	70 - 105 mm Hg
Right Atrial Pressure (RAP)		2 - 6 mm Hg
Right Ventricular Pressure (RVP)	Systolic (RVSP) Diastolic (RVDP)	15 - 25 mm Hg 0 - 8 mm Hg
Pulmonary Artery Pressure (PAP)	Systolic (PASP) Diastolic (PADP)	15 - 25 mm Hg 8 - 15 mm Hg
Mean Pulmonary Artery Pressure (MPAP)	PASP + (2 x PADP)/3	10 - 20 mm Hg
Pulmonary Artery Wedge Pressure (PAWP)		6 - 12 mm Hg
Left Atrial Pressure (LAP)		6 - 12 mm Hg
Cardiac Output (CO)	HR x SV/1000	4.0 - 8.0 L/min
Cardiac Index (CI)	CO/BSA	2.5 - 4.0 -L/min/m2
Stroke Volume (SV)	CO/HR x 1000	60 - 100 ml/beat
Stroke Volume Index (SVI)	CI/HR x 1000	33 - 47 ml/m2/beat
Systemic Vascular Resistance (SVR)	80 x (MAP - RAP) /CO	800 - 1200 dynes•sec/cm5
Systemic Vascular Resistance Index (SVRI)	80 x (MAP - RAP) /CI	1970 - 2390 dynes•sec/cm5/m2
Pulmonary Vascular Resistance (PVR)	80 x (MPAP - PAWP) /CO	<250 dynes• sec/cm5
Pulmonary Vascular Resistance Index (PVRI)	80 x (MPAP - PAWP) /CI	255 - 285 dynes• sec/cm5/m2
Left Ventricular Stroke Work (LVSW)	SV x (MAP - PAWP) x 0.0136	58 - 104 gm-m/beat
Left Ventricular Stroke Work Index (LVSWI)	SVI x (MAP - PAWP) x 0.0136	50 - 62 gm-m/m2/beat
Right Ventricular Stroke Work (RVSW)	SV x (MPAP - RAP) x 0.0136	8 - 16 gm-m/beat
Right Ventricular Stroke Work Index (RVSWI)	SVI x (MPAP - RAP) x 0.0136	5 - 10 gm-m/m2/beat
Coronary Artery Perfusion Pressure (CPP)	Diastolic BP-PAWP	60 - 80 mm Hg
Right Ventricular End-Diastolic Volume (RVEDV)	SV/EF	100 - 160 ml
Right Ventricular End-Systolic Volume (RVESV)	EDV - SV	50 - 100 ml
Right Ventricular Ejection Fraction (RVEF)	SV/EDV	40 - 60%

French Catheter Size Conversion

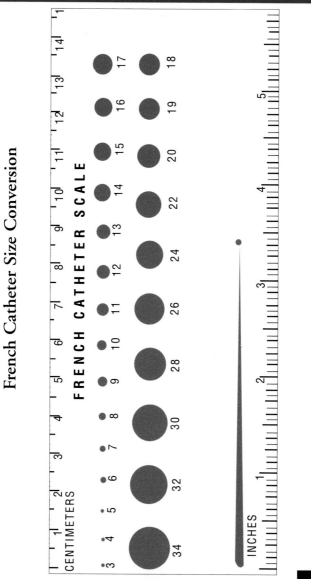

French Catheter Size Conversion

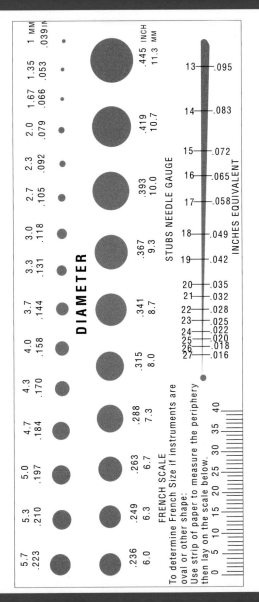

DIAMETER

| 5.7 .223 | 5.3 .210 | 5.0 .197 | 4.7 .184 | 4.3 .170 | 4.0 .158 | 3.7 .144 | 3.3 .131 | 3.0 .118 | 2.7 .105 | 2.3 .092 | 2.0 .079 | 1.67 .066 | 1.35 .053 | 1 MM .039 IN |

| .236 6.0 | .249 6.3 | .263 6.7 | .288 7.3 | .315 8.0 | | .341 8.7 | .367 9.3 | | .393 10.0 | | .419 10.7 | | .445 INCH 11.3 MM |

FRENCH SCALE
To determine French Size if instruments are oval or other shape:
Use strip of paper to measure the periphery then lay on the scale below.

0 5 10 15 20 25 30 35 40

STUBS NEEDLE GAUGE

INCHES EQUIVALENT

13	.095
14	.083
15	.072
16	.065
17	.058
18	.049
19	.042
20	.035
21	.032
22	.028
23	.025
24	.022
25	.020
26	.018
27	.016

References

1. Ahrens TS, Taylor LA. *Hemodynamic Waveform Analysis*. Philadelphia, PA: WB Saunders Co.; 1992.

2. Bridges EJ, Middleton R. Direct Arterial vs. Oscillometric Monitoring of Blood Pressure: Stop Comparing and Pick One (A Decision-Making Algorithm). *Critical Care Nurse*, June 1997, Vol. 17, No. 3, 58-72.

3. Braunwald E (ed.) *Heart Disease A textbook of Cardiovascular Medicine 5th Edition*. W. B. Saunders Co. Philadelphia; 1997.

4. Criley JM, Ross RS. *Cardiovascular Physiology*. Tarpon Springs, Florida:Tampa Tracings; 1971.

5. Daily EK, Schroeder JS. *Techniques in Bedside Hemodynamic Monitoring*. 4th ed. St. Louis: C.V. Mosby; 1989.

6. Dantzker DR, *Cardiopulmonary Critical Care*. 2nd ed. Philadelphia, PA, W.B.Saunders Co; 1991.

7. Darovic GO. *Hemodynamic Monitoring: Invasive and Noninvasive Clinical Application*. 2nd ed. Philadelphia, PA: W.B. Saunders Co.; 1995.

8. Diebel L, Wilson RF, Heins J, et al. End-Diastolic Volume Versus Pulmonary Artery Wedge Pressure in Evaluating Cardiac Preload in Trauma Patients. *The Journal of Trauma*, 1994, Vol 37, No 6, 950-955.

9. Durham R, Neunaber K, Volger G, et al., et al, Right Ventricular End-Diastolic Volume as a Measure of Preload. *The Journal of Trauma: Injury, Infection, and Critical Care*, 1995, Vol 39, No 2, 218-224.

10. Halfman-Franey M, Bergstrom D. Clinical Management Using Direct and Derived Parameters. *Critical Care Nursing Clinics of North America*, September 1989, Vol 1, No. 3; 547-561.

11. Hazinski MF, Cummins RO (eds). 1996 *Handbook of Emergency Cardiac Care for Healthcare Providers*. Dallas: American Heart Association; 1996.

12. Headley JM. Strategies to Optimize the Cardiorespiratory Status of the Critically Ill. *AACN Clinical Issues in Critical Care Nursing*. 1995:6(1);121-134.

13. Headley JM. *Invasive Hemodynamic Monitoring: Physiological Principles and Clinical Applications*. Irvine, CA.: Baxter Healthcare Corporation: 1989.

14. Hensley FA, Martin DE (eds). *A Practical Approach to Cardiac Anesthesia*. 2nd ed., Boston: Little, Brown and CO; 1995.

15. Ivanov RI, Calvin JE, Parrillo JE, Liebson PR. Pulmonary Artery Catheterization: A Balanced Look at the Controversy. *The Journal of Critical Illness*, August 1997, Vol 12, No 8, 469-476.

16. Kaplan JA (ed). *Cardiac Anesthesia* 2nd. Ed. Orlando: Grune & Stratton Inc; 1987.

17. Kirby RR, Taylor RW, Civetta JM. *Handbook of Critical Care*. Philadelphia: J.B. Lippincott Co; 1994.

18. Lichtenthal PR, Wade LD. Continuous Cardiac Output Measurements. *J Cardiothorac Vasc Anesth*. 1994:8(6); 668-670.

19. Lichtenthal PR, Collins JT. Multipurpose pulmonary artery catheter. *Ann Thorac Surg*. 1983:36(4):493.

20. Lumb PD, Bryan-Brown CW. *Complications in Critical Care Medicine*. Chicago; Year Book Medical Publishers, Inc.; 1988.

21. Martin L. *Pulmonary Physiology in Clinical Practice: The Essentials for Patient Care and Evaluation*. St. Louis: The C.V. Mosby Co; 1987.

22. Opie LH (ed.). *Drugs for the Heart*. 2nd ed., Philadelphia: W.B. Saunders CO: 1987.

23. Perret C, Tagan D, Feihl F, Marini JJ. *The Pulmonary Artery Catheter in Critical Care: A Concise Handbook*. Cambridge, Blackwell Science Inc; 1996.

24. Pinsky MR (ed). *Applied Cardiovascular Physiology*. New York, NY, Springer;1997.

25. Ryan TJ, Anderson JL, Antman EM, et. al., ACC/AHA Guidelines for the Management of Patients With Acute Myocardial Infarction: Executive Summary. *Circulation*, November 1, 1996; 94, (9):2341-2350.

26. Sharkey SW, *A Guide to Interpretation of Hemodynamic Data in the Coronary Care Unit*. Philadelphia: Lippincott-Raven; 1997.

27. Sprung CL (ed). *The Pulmonary Artery Catheter: Methodology and Clinical Applications*. 2nd ed. Closter, NJ: Critical Care Research Associates, Inc.; 1993.

28. *Stedman's Medical Dictionary*. Baltimore: Williams & Wilkins; 1995.

29. Taylor RW (ed). Controversies in Pulmonary Artery Catheterization. *New Horizons*. 1997: 5(3); 173-296.

30. Wilson RF. *Critical Care Manual: Applied Physiology and Principles of Therapy*. 2nd ed. Philadelphia: FA Davis Co; 1992.

31. Woods SL, Froelicher ESS, Halpenny CJ, et al. *Cardiac Nursing*. 3rd ed. Philadelphia: JB Lippincott Co; 1995.

REFERENCES